AF559646

Poultry Production and Management

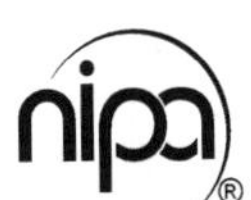

NIPA® GENX ELECTRONIC RESOURCES & SOLUTIONS P. LTD.
New Delhi-110 034

Poultry Production and Management

Rafiqul Islam
Assistant Professor
Department of Poultry Science, College of Veterinary Science
Assam Agricultural University, Khanapara, Guwahati-781022, Assam, India

Arfan Ali
Associate Professor
Department of Veterinary Microbiology, College of Veterinary Science
Assam Agricultural University, Khanapara, Guwahati-781022, Assam, India

Mihir Sarma
Scientist (Poultry)
Directorate of Research (Veterinary)
Assam Agricultural University, Khanapara, Guwahati-781022, Assam, India

Pankaj Deka
Assistant Professor-cum-Virologist
Department of Veterinary Microbiology, College of Veterinary Science
Assam Agricultural University, Khanapara, Guwahati-781022, Assam, India

Mustafizur Rahman
Assistant Professor
Department of Animal Husbandry & Dairying
SCS College of Agriculture, Assam Agricultural University
Rangamati, Dhubri, Assam, India

Ashim Kumar Saikia
Associate Professor
Department of Animal Nutrition
Lakhimpur College of Veterinary Science
Assam Agricultural University, Joyhing, North Lakhimpur, Assam, India

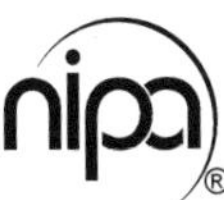

NIPA® GENX ELECTRONIC RESOURCES & SOLUTIONS P. LTD.
New Delhi-110 034

NIPA® GENX ELECTRONIC RESOURCES & SOLUTIONS P. LTD.

101,103, Vikas Surya Plaza, CU Block
L.S.C. Market, Pitam Pura, New Delhi-110 034
Ph : +91-11-43860225, Mob.: +91 9717133558, 9540816132
E-mail: newindiapublishingagency@gmail.com
Website: www.nipaersources.com

Print ISBN: 978-93-58879-92-6
ebook ISBN: 978-93-58879-94-0

NIPA® also publishes books in a variety of electronic formats. Some content that appears in print may not be available in electronic books, and vice versa.

Composed and Designed by NIPA®.

Preface

Poultry has emerged as one of the most dynamic and impactful segments of Indian agriculture, advancing on the strength of improved commercial strains, rising disposable incomes, expanding food-service channels, and better distribution and delivery networks. Together, these forces have reshaped demand for eggs and poultry meat and positioned the sector as a vital contributor to nutrition and livelihoods.

Beyond its market momentum, poultry supports a wide spectrum of jobs and enterprises—from hatcheries and feed mills to veterinary services, research and development, and retail—while reinforcing rural economies and food security.

At the same time, indigenous and backyard systems remain central to the rural ecosystem, providing low-cost animal protein, supplemental income, and efficient waste conversion—especially for women and youth engaged in household poultry.

This book, ***"Poultry Production and Management"***, has been developed to bridge foundational science and field practice. It opens with India's industry backdrop and growth drivers, then moves to breeds and breed standards, highlighting the commercial importance of White Leghorn for layers and Cornish-based broilers, with ready-reference tables on strain performance.

Subsequent chapters walk through breeding as a scientific enterprise—covering systems, selection and culling, and practical judging cues—so that readers can align genetic improvement with measurable gains in meat and egg productivity.

Recognizing on-farm realities, the text consolidates day-to-day management for broilers and layers, breeder flock standards, and robust disease-prevention checklists, bringing vaccination, deworming, litter care, and biosecurity into one accessible toolkit.

It also introduces integration and contract farming models that now characterize much of commercial broiler production, clarifying roles, inputs, and payout logic for growers within coordinated value chains.

We have not shied away from the sector's constraints. Rising input costs, disease risks, import competition, and uneven biosecurity standards are treated not only as challenges but as design constraints for resilient operations, guiding the reader toward cost-aware rations, disciplined health protocols, and farm-level risk management. In parallel, the book foregrounds India's rich indigenous avian biodiversity and the socio-economic value of native and improved backyard birds, encouraging context-specific strategies that balance productivity with cultural and ecological fit.

Our intended audience includes undergraduate and postgraduate students in veterinary and animal sciences, extension personnel, entrepreneurs, and progressive farmers. Throughout, we have emphasized clarity, comparative tables, and practice-ready checklists to make the material useful both in classrooms and on farms. We gratefully acknowledge the many teachers, practitioners, and farm families whose insight and experience ground these pages.

We hope this work helps readers translate sound science into profitable, ethical, and biosecure poultry enterprises—enterprises that nourish people, create dignified employment, and steward India's diverse avian resources for the long term.

Authors

Contents

1

Introduction to Poultry Industry and Its Development in India

Rafiqul Islam and Arfan Ali

History of poultry production

Domestication of birds has a long history, with evidence of their existence and use dating back thousands of years. Here are some key points:

- **Chickens:** Archaeological evidence suggests domesticated chickens existed in China 8,000 years ago and later spread to Western Europe, possibly via Russia. The cockfighting in India 3,000 years ago indicates their cultural significance. Modern domestic chickens (*Gallus domesticus*) evolved from the wild red jungle fowl (*Gallus gallus*), native to India and Southeast Asia.
- **Pigeons:** The domestic pigeon (*Columba liviaf. domestica*) is considered the world's oldest domesticated bird.
- **Geese:** Domestic geese (*Anseranserdomesticus* in Africa, Europe, and West Asia; *Ansercygnoides* in East Asia) were domesticated in Egypt over 4,000 years ago and have significance in Roman mythology.
- **Other Poultry:**
  - Guinea fowl (*Numida meleagris*) in Africa
  - Muscovy duck (*Cairinamoschata*) in Central and South America
  - Domestic turkey (*Meleagris gallopavo*) from Mexico
  - Mallard duck (*Anas platyrhynchos*) likely domesticated in Southeast Asia
  - Ratites, including ostrich, emu, and rhea, are among the latest domesticated poultry species.
- **Historical Spread:** Initially domesticated birds were used in religious rituals and were spread westward from India to Greece and Western Europe, notably by Roman armies, who used them for meat and eggs.
- **Introduction to North America:** The first European settlers brought chickens with them.

- **Early Chicken Rearing:** Initially carried out by women and children, with low productivity (about 30 eggs per annum) dependent on favorable seasons.
- **19th Century:** Chicken breeding became a hobby, focusing on colorful feathered breeds. Improved incubators in the late 19th century led to commercial breeding for egg and meat production.
- **20th Century:** Emphasis on poultry nutrition and industrialization led to automated, large-scale farming. Chicken production is now highly organized in India, comprising about 80% of the livestock market value.

These points outline the rich history and evolution of poultry domestication and its impact on human culture and agriculture.

Importance of poultry farming in India

Poultry farming is essential in India, significantly contributing to nutrition, employment, and economic development. It provides affordable, nutritious food to combat malnutrition, especially in rural areas, and generates millions of jobs. The sector supports 30 million backyard poultry farmers and continues to grow due to urbanization and changing food habits. Technological advancements have improved productivity, and poultry farming produces valuable organic fertilizer. Chicken dominates the market, accounting for a major portion of egg and meat production in the country.

- **Nutritional Impact:** Over 75% of Indians live in rural areas, many suffering from deficiency diseases like anemia. Poultry eggs and meat, being nutritious and affordable, can help combat malnutrition.
- **Employment:** The sector offers direct employment to over 1 million broiler farmers and 25,000 layer farmers, plus 5 million indirect jobs. Each increase in egg and meat consumption creates additional job opportunities.
- **Economic Support:** Backyard poultry farming supports around 30 million farmers, providing supplemental income and nutrition.
- **Growth Potential**: Poultry production and consumption are predicted to rise due to changing food habits, urbanization, and increased nutrition awareness.
- **Technological Advancements:** The sector has seen rapid growth through new technologies, including improved chicken incubators, high-yielding layers (310-340 eggs per year), and broilers (2.4-2.6 kg at 6 weeks). Advancements in nutrition, housing, management, and disease control have also contributed to increase productivity.

- **Organic Fertilizer:** Poultry farming produces 6.25-8.0 million tons of poultry manure annually, used as organic fertilizer (The Hindu, 9th October, 2009).
- **Market Share:** Poultry meat constitutes about 45% of total meat consumption, with chicken dominating at 95% of egg production.

These factors accentuate the significant impact of poultry farming on India's nutrition, employment, and economic development.

Overview of Poultry Production in India

Poultry production in India is a vital sector catering to the production of eggs and meat, crucial for meeting dietary demands. Here are key insights:

- Poultry encompasses various domesticated birds, including chicken, duck, and quail, reared primarily for egg and meat production.
- India's poultry population totals 851.81 million, with 62.78% farmed commercially and 37.22% in backyard systems.
- In 2022-23, India produced 138.38 billion eggs, ranking second globally, with a per capita availability of 101 eggs annually.
- Poultry meat production contributes significantly, totaling 4.995 million tonnes annually, representing 51.14% of the country's total meat production.
- Andhra Pradesh leads in egg production, followed by Tamil Nadu, Telangana, and others.
- Annual broiler meat production is estimated at 5 million tonnes, positioning India fifth globally.
- The Indian poultry market reached INR 2099.2 billion in 2023, projected to grow at a CAGR of 8.1% to reach USD 61.41 billion by 2032.
- Bridging production gaps is critical to meet increasing demand.
- Key poultry markets include Maharashtra, Tamil Nadu, Andhra Pradesh, among others.
- India exported 664,753.46 MT of poultry products worth INR 1,081.62 crores during 2022-23, with major destinations being Oman, Indonesia, and the UAE.

This comprehensive overview underscores India's pivotal role in global poultry production and its potential for robust expansion in the years ahead.

Global Poultry Production Scenario

Poultry production globally is a cornerstone of the agriculture industry, pivotal in meeting global demands for both eggs and meat. Here's a comprehensive look at the current landscape:

- **Egg Production:** In 2022, global egg production soared to 1,627 trillion eggs, with China alone accounting for 37% of the total, underscoring its dominance in the market.
- **Chicken Meat Production:** Forecasted to reach 103.4 million metric tons in 2023, global chicken meat production reflects robust growth, primarily driven by expansions in Brazil and the United States. Despite challenges such as fluctuating feed prices, advancements in production technologies have bolstered output in many regions.
- **Global Production Leaders:** China solidified its position as the largest producer of poultry meat since 2021, producing over 15% of the world's total, closely followed by the United States and Brazil. This dominance underscores China's strategic importance in global poultry markets.
- **Regional Dynamics:** Asia remains a powerhouse, contributing more than 64% of the world's eggs in 2021. The region's significant production capabilities are bolstered by diverse farming practices and increasing consumption patterns. In 2021, a total of 70.66 billion birds were produced/slaughtered globally, with Asia accounting for nearly half or almost 33 billion chickens.
- **Production Trends:** While meat production is rising in the United States, it has stabilized in China. The increase in white feather broilers has compensated for the decrease in yellow feather broiler production in 2023, highlighting China's adaptive strategies in poultry farming.
- **Export Trends:** The Netherlands emerges as a pivotal player in global poultry exports, exporting 351,223 tonnes of eggs in 2021 and substantial quantities of chicken meat. Benefitting from favorable trade agreements within Europe, the Netherlands continues to expand its market reach.
- **Global Trade Dynamics:** Global poultry exports are projected to increase marginally by 1% in 2023, totaling 13.7 million tons. Brazil anticipates a notable 7% export growth, driven by its avian influenza-free status and expansive market access.
- **Ukrainian Impact:** Ukraine has capitalized on European free-trade measures post-Russian invasion, significantly boosting its chicken meat exports to European markets. This strategic maneuver has positioned Ukraine as a key player in the global poultry trade.
- **Import Trends:** Hong Kong emerges as a significant importer of eggs, driven by high demand and a dense population. This demand underscores global poultry's critical role in meeting diverse dietary needs across densely populated urban centers.

This comprehensive overview emphasizes the dynamic nature of global poultry production, shaped by regional strengths, trade dynamics, and technological advancements. As the industry continues to evolve, these insights provide a robust foundation for understanding its global impact and future prospects.

Employment Opportunities in the Poultry Industry

The poultry sector offers diverse employment opportunities across various sectors, playing a crucial role in rural development and economic growth. Here's a comprehensive overview:

1. **Farm-Level Employment:** Poultry farms employ workers for essential tasks such as feeding, watering, cleaning, and maintaining poultry houses. Skilled workers are also hired for breeding, vaccination, and overall flock management.
2. **Contract Farming:** Large poultry companies engage in contract farming, providing inputs, technical support, and market access to contract farmers. This model not only creates jobs for farmers but also supports ancillary services such as feed suppliers, veterinary care, and transportation.
3. **Processing and Manufacturing:** The poultry industry features a substantial processing and manufacturing sector encompassing poultry meat processing plants and egg grading and packaging facilities. These operations rely on a skilled workforce for meat processing, quality control, packaging, labeling, and distribution. This sector plays a crucial role in ensuring the efficient processing and delivery of poultry products to consumers worldwide.
4. **Supply Chain and Logistics:** Employment opportunities exist in the supply chain and logistics sector, including transportation of poultry products from farms to processing plants, distribution to retail outlets, and export logistics. Roles encompass drivers, logistics coordinators, warehouse staff, and distribution personnel.
5. **Retail and Marketing:** Poultry products are distributed through various retail channels, including supermarkets, grocery stores, and specialized poultry shops. These outlets require employees for sales, customer service, inventory management, and marketing activities.
6. **Veterinary and Healthcare Services:** The poultry industry creates demand for veterinary services to ensure the health and well-being of poultry flocks. Veterinarians, veterinary assistants, and animal health professionals are employed to provide healthcare, disease prevention, and treatment services to poultry farms.

7. **Research and Development:** Employment opportunities in research and development involve scientists, researchers, and technical experts studying poultry nutrition, genetics, disease management, and technological advancements. Their work aims to improve production efficiency and address industry challenges.
8. **Supporting Industries:** The poultry industry stimulates employment in supporting sectors such as feed manufacturing, equipment suppliers, packaging materials, and pharmaceuticals. These industries offer jobs in manufacturing, sales, marketing, and distribution, supporting the overall poultry supply chain.

The poultry industry's employment impact extends beyond direct roles, contributing to economic stability and improving livelihoods in rural communities. It serves as a cornerstone of agricultural economies worldwide, supporting local and global food security while fostering innovation and sustainability.

Major Growth Drivers of the Poultry Industry in India

The poultry industry in India is driven by several key factors that contribute to its growth and expansion:

- **Introduction of Hybrid Chickens:** Adoption of newly developed hybrid chicken breeds such as Ross, Cobb, Shaver, Babcock, and Hyaline, known for faster growth, high survivability rates, excellent Feed Conversion Ratio (FCR), and enhanced profitability.
- **Rising Disposable Incomes:** Increasing disposable incomes and per capita consumption levels, leading to higher demand for poultry products.
- **Expansion of Food Services Market:** Growth in the food services sector, including restaurants, hotels, and catering services, which drive demand for poultry meat and eggs.
- **Population Growth:** India's growing population continues to boost demand for affordable & nutritious protein sources like poultry products.
- **Increased Health Awareness:** Rising health consciousness among consumers, leading to a preference for lean protein sources and nutritious foods.
- **Growing Consumption of Protein-based Foods:** Increasing awareness of the health benefits associated with protein-rich diets, further driving demand for poultry products.

- **Development of Distribution Networks:** Strengthening of distribution channels and logistics networks, ensuring efficient supply chain management from farms to consumers.
- **Utilization of Online Food Delivery Channels:** Growing utilization of online platforms such as Zomato, Uber Eats, Swiggy, and others for food ordering, expanding accessibility and convenience in accessing poultry products.

These factors collectively contribute to the dynamic growth and sustainability of India's poultry industry, positioning it as a vital sector in the country's agricultural and economic landscape.

Table 1.1: Some of the Leading Companies/Startups Involved in Poultry Industry in India:

Sl. No.	Name of the company	Head Quarter
Major poultry integrators		
1.	Suguna Foods Private Ltd.	Coimbatore, Tamil Nadu
2.	Godrej Agrovet Ltd.	Mumbai, Maharashtra
3.	Indian Broiler Group	Rajnandagaon, Chhattisgarh
4.	Pioneer Poultry Group	Coimbatore, Tamil Nadu
5.	RM Hatcheries	Panipat, Haryana
6.	Simran Farms Ltd.	Indore, Madhya Pradesh
7.	Skylark Hatcheries Pvt. Ltd,	Jind, Haryana
8.	Venky's (India) Ltd.	Pune, Maharashtra
9.	Srinivasa Farms	Hyderabad, Telangana
10.	Sneha Poultry	Hyderabad, Telangana
Major poultry feed manufacturers/supplier		
1.	Suguna Foods Private Ltd.	Coimbatore, Tamil Nadu
2.	JapfaComfeeds India Pvt. Ltd. (Japfa Ltd)	Pune, Maharashtra
3.	Venkateswara Hatcheries Pvt. Ltd.	Pune, Maharashtra
4.	Anmol feeds Pvt. Ltd.	Patna, Bihar
5.	Godrej Agrovet Limited (Godrej Industries Ltd.)	Mumbai, Maharashtra
6.	SKM Animal Feeds and Foods (India) Pvt. Ltd.	Bengaluru, Karnataka
7.	Cargill Incorporated	Bengaluru, Karnataka
8.	Amrit Group KSE Ltd.	Kolkata
9.	Kapila Krishi Udyog Ltd.	Kanpur, UP
10.	Avanti Feeds Ltd.	Hyderabad, Telangana

Major poultry equipment manufacturer/supplier		
1.	Dhumal Industries India Pvt. Ltd.	Nashik, Maharashtra
2.	Supreme Equipment	Nashik, Maharashtra
3.	Mayura Industries	Coimbatore, TN
4.	Krishna Polyplast	Bharuch, Gujarat
5.	Karamsar Poultry Appliances	Mayapuri, New Delhi
6.	Poultry India	Ghaziabad, UP
7.	Vinayak Poultry	Karnal, Haryana
8.	Vijay Raj Poultry Equipment Pvt. Ltd.	Hyderabad, Telangana
9.	Chakra Poultry Equipment	Hyderabad, Telangana
Major animal health care companies		
1.	Zoetis India Limited	Mumbai, Maharashtra
2.	Virbac Animal Health India Pvt. Ltd.	Mumbai, Maharashtra
3.	Elanco India Pvt. Ltd.	Gurgaon, Haryana
4.	Merck Animal Health India	Multinational
5.	Indian Immunologicals Ltd.	Hyderabad, Telangana
6.	Intas Pharmaceuticals Ltd. (Animal Health Div.)	Ahmedabad, Gujarat
7.	Bayer Animal Health	Multinational
8.	Venky's (India) Ltd.	Pune, India
9.	Hester Biosciences Ltd.	Ahmedabad, Gujarat
10.	Biovet Private Ltd.	Bengaluru, Karnataka
Leading Startups in Poultry Industry		**Founded in**
1.	Licious	2015
2.	Fresh to Home	2015
3.	Nando's	2016
4.	Zappfresh	2015
5.	Captain Fresh	2019
6.	Tender Cuts	2016
7.	Eggoz	2017
8.	Happy Hens	2017

Challenges of Poultry Production in India

The poultry industry in India faces several challenges that impact its operations and growth:

- **Higher Cost of Inputs:** Rising costs of inputs such as feeds and logistics increase production expenses, affecting profitability for poultry farmers.
- **High Risk of Disease Outbreaks like Avian Influenza (Bird flu):** Poultry farms are susceptible to disease outbreaks, which can lead to significant economic losses and disruptions in production.

- **Competition from International Markets:** Indian poultry producers contend with competition from cheaper imports and fluctuating international market dynamics, affecting domestic pricing and market share.
- **Insufficient Bio-Security Standards:** Inadequate bio-security measures among poultry keepers increase the risk of disease transmission within and between farms, posing health threats to poultry stocks.
- **Enviromental stress:** Majority of the poultry birds are housed in open sheds/farms without any control of shed enviroment, exposing birds to various enviromental stress and potenial diseases.

2

Poultry Breeds Their Standards and Performances

Arfan Ali and Rafiqul Islam

Genetic Classification of Poultry

Understanding the genetic classification of poultry is essential for breeders and farmers to optimize the performance and standards of different commercial breeds. Here's a detailed overview:

Evolutionary Background

- In the process of evolution, cold-blooded (poikilothermic) reptiles are considered the ancestors of birds.
- Birds are warm-blooded (homeothermic) feathered creatures adapted for hot and dry climates in their terrestrial habitats.

Chromosomal Categories

- **Sex Chromosomes:** Carry genetic material that determines the sex of an offspring.
- **Autosomes:** Non-sex chromosomes that carry the bulk of genetic information.

Genetic Material

- **DNA (Deoxyribonucleic Acid):** The genetic material containing the instructions for the development and function of an organism, arranged in double helix-shaped strands.
- **Gene:** A segment of DNA that provides the blueprint for a cell's function and ultimately determines specific characteristics of an organism.

Chromosomes and Genes

- Genes come in pairs, with each parent contributing one gene to each pair. The phenotype (observable trait) of a chicken depends on the gene pair composition.

- **Homozygous:** Both genes in a pair are identical.
- **Heterozygous:** The genes in a pair are different.

Avian Karyotype

- Most avian karyotypes include chromosomes of varying lengths, termed macro- and microchromosomes, making bird karyotypes distinct from those of mammals.
- The chicken karyotype consists of 78 chromosomes (2n = 78), including 38 pairs of autosomes and one pair of sex chromosomes. Females are the heterogametic sex (ZW), and males are the homogametic sex (ZZ).

Sex Chromosomes in Chickens

- In chickens, the sex chromosomes are referred to as Z and W, whereas in humans they are X and Y.
- Female chickens are heterogametic (ZW), meaning they have both types of sex chromosomes.
- Male chickens are homogametic (ZZ), meaning they have two of the same type of sex chromosomes.
- Conversely, in humans, females are homogametic (XX), and males are heterogametic (XY).

Understanding these genetic principles is crucial for managing poultry breeding programs and improving the performance and standards of commercial poultry breeds.

Table 2.1: Genus and species of different domesticated fowls with their chromosome number

Sl. No.	Common Name	Zoological Name	Chromosome Nos.
1	Chicken	Gallus gallusdomesticus	78
2	Japanese quail	Coturnix coturnix japonica	78
3	Bobwhite quail	Colinus virginianus	78
4	Guinea fowl	Numida meleagris	78
5	Duck	Anas platyrynchos	80
6	Muscovy Duck	Cairinamoschata	80
7	Rhea	Rhea americana	80
8	Turkey	Meleagris gallopavo	80
9	Goose	Anseranser	80
10	Partridge	Perdix perdix	80
11	Pheasant	Phasianuscolchicus	82
12	Emu	Dromaius novaehollandiae	82
13	Pea fowl	Pavo cristatus	80
14	Ostrich	Struthio camelus	80
15	Pigeon	Columba livia	80
16	Dove	Columba oenas	80
17	African Parrot	Psittacus erithacus	62-64
18	Indian Parrot	Lovius rotates	80
19	Budgerigar	Melopsittacus undulates	26

Table 2.2: Nomenclature of different poultry species

Sl. No.	Species	Male	Adult Female	Young			
				0-8 weeks		9-18 weeks	
				Male	Female	Male	Female
1	Chicken	Cock	Hen	Chick		Cockerel	Pullet
2	Duck	Drake	Duck	Drakeling	Duckling	Drakelet	Ducklet
3	Goose	Gander	Goose	Gosling		-	-
4	Turkey	Tom Turkey	Turkey hen	Poult	Poult	-	-
5	Quail	Cock	Hen	Chick	Chick	-	-
6	Pigeon	Cock	Hen	Squab	Squab	-	-
7	Guinea Fowl	Cock	Hen	Keet	Keet	-	-
8	Pheasant	Cock	Hen	Chick	Chick	-	-
9	Partridge	Cock	Hen	Chick	Chick	-	-
10	Swan	Cob	Pen	Cygnet	Cygnet	-	-

Table 2.2: Definitions and Terms related to poultry

Species	Term	Definition
Chicken	Cockerel	A young male chicken, typically 9 to 18 weeks old.
Chicken	Pullet	A young female chicken, typically 9 to 18 weeks old.
Duck	Drakeling	A young male duck, typically 0 to 8 weeks old.
Duck	Duckling	A young female duck, typically 0 to 8 weeks old.
Duck	Drakelet	A young male duck, typically 9 to 18 weeks old.
Duck	Ducklet	A young female duck, typically 9 to 18 weeks old.
Goose	Gosling	A young goose, both male and female, 0 to 8 weeks old.
Turkey	Poult	A young turkey, both male and female, 0 to 8 weeks old.
Quail	Chick	A young quail, both male and female, 0 to 8 weeks old.
Pigeon	Squab	A young pigeon, both male and female, 0 to 8 weeks old.
Guinea Fowl	Keet	A young guinea fowl, both male and female, 0 to 8 weeks old.
Pheasant	Chick	A young pheasant, both male and female, 0 to 8 weeks old.
Partridge	Chick	A young partridge, both male and female, 0 to 8 weeks old.
Swan	Cygnet	A young swan, both male and female, 0 to 8 weeks old.

This detailed classification aids in precise identification and management of poultry across various species, ensuring effective communication and operational efficiency within the poultry industry.

Classification of Chickens

Class: The term “class” designates a group of birds developed in certain regions or geographical areas.e.g.American, Asiatic, Mediterranean, English etc.

Breed: A breed is a group of chickens that have a phenotype or appearance, characteristics, and/or behavior that distinguish them from other chickens of the same class. Breeds possess distinctive shapes, conformations, plumage colors, comb types, general body weights, and are true to breed.e.g. Aseel, Rhode Island Red, Leghorn, Cornish.

Variety: The term “variety” is used to sub-classify breeds. Varieties within a breed can be differentiated by plumage color, pattern, and comb type. e.g. White Leghorn, Black Leghorn, Brown Leghorn, Barred Plymouth Rock.

Strain: Strains are sub-classifications of a breed, typically named after the person who developed them or the research station. They are developed with an emphasis on specific traits such as egg production, early maturity, better feed efficiency, and egg weight. e.g. Meyer strain of White Leghorn, Forsgate strain of White Leghorn.

Lines: These are sub-classes of strains used for the production of commercial hybrids. e.g. Male line, Female line, Body weight line, Egg production line.

This hierarchical classification helps in the systematic breeding, management, and research of poultry, facilitating better understanding and advancement in poultry science.

General Characteristics of Various Standard Classes of Chicken

a. American Class

- **Characteristics:**
  - Medium to heavy-sized birds, primarily meant for meat or brown egg production.
  - Clean yellow shanks and yellow skin (except Jersey Black Giant, where the shanks are black).
  - Red ear lobes and rose or single combs.
  - **Examples:** Plymouth Rock, Wyandotte, Rhode Island Red, Jersey Black Giant, New Hampshire.

b. Asiatic Class

- **Characteristics:**
  - Heavy in size, and poor layers.
  - Lay brown eggs.
  - Broody with a motherly instinct.
  - Red ear lobes.
  - Mostly have feathered yellow shanks and yellow skin (except Langshan).
  - **Examples:** Brahma, Cochin, Langshan.

c. English Class

- **Characteristics:**
  - Medium to large-sized birds.
  - Single comb (except Cornish with pea comb), red ear lobes.
  - White skin (except Cornish where it is yellow), clean and white shank (except Australorp, where it is dark slate and in Cornish where it is yellow).
  - Lay brown shell eggs (except Dorking, which lays white shelled eggs).
  - **Examples:** Australorp, Cornish, Dorking, Orpington, Sussex.

d. Mediterranean Class

- **Characteristics:**
  - Small size, egg-type, non-broody.
  - White ear lobes, yellow or white skin.
  - Clean and yellow/slate-colored shanks and lay white-shelled eggs.
  - **Examples:** Leghorn, Minorca, Ancona, Andalusian.

Important Facts about Chicken Breeds

- **Jersey Giant:**
  - Largest chicken breed in the world, belonging to the American class.
  - Standard adult weight:
  - Male: 13 pounds (5.90 kg)
  - **Female:** 10 pounds (4.5 kg)
- **Serama:**
  - Smallest chicken breed in the world.
  - Originated in Malaysia.
  - Adult size ranges from 7 oz (198.66 g) to 19 oz (539.22 g).
- **Brahma:**
  - Largest breed in the Asiatic class.
- **Cornish:**
  - Largest breed in the English class.
- **Varieties:**
  - Each breed of chicken has different varieties, except Australorp and Andalusian.
- **Feather Color Patterns:**
  - Wyandotte, Langshan, Australorp, Hamburg, and Polish breeds have a variety of attractive feather color patterns.
- **Behavioral Traits:**
  - New Hampshire Red breed is aggressive.
  - Plymouth Rock breed is docile and tame.

Additional Facts of Academic Importance

- **Egg Production:**
  - The Leghorn breed, belonging to the Mediterranean class, is one of the most prolific layers, with some hens capable of laying over 300 eggs per year.
- **Genetics:**
  - Chickens were the first domesticated animals to have their genome sequenced. The sequencing of the chicken genome has provided valuable insights into avian biology and evolution.
- **Growth Rates:**
  - Modern broiler chickens are bred for rapid growth and can reach market weight in as little as six weeks. This contrasts sharply with traditional breeds, which may take several months to reach the same weight.
- **Dual-Purpose Breeds:**
  - Some breeds, like the Rhode Island Red, are considered dual-purpose because they are good for both egg and meat production. This makes them valuable for small-scale and backyard poultry farming.
- **Nutritional Contributions:**
  - Eggs from different breeds can vary in nutritional content. For example, the Araucana breed lays eggs that are naturally higher in omega-3 fatty acids.
- **Behavioral Studies:**
  - Chickens have been used extensively in behavioral studies. They are known for their complex social structures and have been observed to exhibit behaviors such as empathy and problem-solving.
- **Heat Tolerance:**
  - Some breeds are better adapted to hot climates. For example, the Naked Neck breed, also known as the Turken, has fewer feathers, which helps it stay cool in hot weather.
- **Disease Resistance:**
  - Certain indigenous breeds, like the Aseel from India, are known for their resilience and resistance to diseases, making them valuable in low-input systems where veterinary care might be limited.

- **Historical Significance:**
    - The domestication of chicken dates back to over 8,000 years ago in Southeast Asia. Chickens have played a significant role in human culture, economy, and diet throughout history.
- **Economic Impact:**
    - The poultry industry is a major contributor to global agriculture, providing a significant portion of the world's protein supply. It is also a major source of employment and income in many countries.

These facts highlight the diverse and significant roles that chickens and the poultry industry play in agriculture, science, and society.

Table 2.3: Some important breeds of chicken with their characteristic features

Parameter	**Leghorn**	**Rhode Island Red**	**New Hampshire**	**Australorp**	**Light Sussex**
Origin	Leghorn village of Italy. Breed of Mediterranean class.	Rhode Island state of America. Breed of American class.	New Hampshire state of America. Developed from RIR.	Australia. Developed from Black Orpington (English breed).	Sussex county of England. Light variety of Sussex breed of English class.
General Appearance	Small and compact, small head with well set comb and wattle, long back, prominent breast, tail lowered down, neatest of all birds.	Long rectangular body, broad and deep breast, flat back, massive look.	Less rectangular than RIR.	Very fleshy, body slopes towards tail, deep body, closely feathered, long back, upright, less massive look.	Deep body with good fleshing quality, broad shoulder.
Plumage Colour	White evenly distributed over the entire body.	Brownish red and well glossed. Black tail feathers and sickle feathers (in male). Slight black marking at the base of the neck feathers (in females).	Chestnut red. Black main tail feathers. Lower neck feathers in females are distinctly tipped with black.	Black, plumage is lustrous greenish black in all sections of the body.	White plumage with black streaked feathers on neck and tail.
Standard Weight (Adult)	Cock: 2.7 kg Hen: 2.0 kg	Cock: 3.8 kg Hen: 3.0 kg	Cock: 3.8 kg Hen: 3.0 kg	Cock: 3.8 kg Hen: 3.0 kg	Cock: 4.0 kg Hen: 3.0 kg
Skin Colour	Yellow	Yellow	Yellow	White	White
Colour of Earlobe	Yellowish white	Reddish	Reddish	Red	Red

Plumage Colour	White evenly distributed over the entire body.	Brownish red and well glossed. Black tail feathers and sickle feathers (in male). Slight black marking at the base of the neck feathers (in females).	Chestnut red. Black main tail feathers. Lower neck feathers in females are distinctly tipped with black.	Black, plumage is lustrous greenish black in all sections of the body.	White plumage with black streaked feathers on neck and tail.
Standard Weight (Adult)	Cock: 2.7 kg Hen: 2.0 kg	Cock: 3.8 kg Hen: 3.0 kg	Cock: 3.8 kg Hen: 3.0 kg	Cock: 3.8 kg Hen: 3.0 kg	Cock: 4.0 kg Hen: 3.0 kg
Skin Colour	Yellow	Yellow	Yellow	White	White
Colour of Earlobe	Yellowish white	Reddish	Reddish	Red	Red
Shank	Yellow coloured, clean	Yellow coloured, clean	Yellow, clean	Black or dark slate coloured, clean	White coloured, clean
Colour of Beak	Yellow	Blackish	Yellow	Black	Coloured
Egg Shell Colour	White	Brown	Brown	Brown	Brown
Commercial Importance	Egg type bird. All commercial hybrid layers derived from this breed.	Dual purpose for egg and meat. More disease resistant than other exotic breeds. Used for upgrading local/desi stock.	Dual purpose for egg and meat.	Dual purpose for egg and meat. Can maintain themselves in wet and heavy rainfall areas.	Meat type.

This table organizes the key parameters for each breed, making it easy to compare their characteristics and commercial importance.

Commercial Strains of Broilers and Layers

The poultry industry utilizes various commercial strains of broilers and layers to optimize production. The White Leghorn is a popular breed for commercial layer production, while the Cornish breed is crucial for developing different commercial broiler strains. The performances of these strains can vary significantly due to differences in their genetic makeup.

Table 2.4: Some Common Commercial Broiler and Layer Strains

Sl. No.	Broiler strains	Layer strains
1	Ross	BV-300 (White)
2	Arbor Acre	BV-380 (Brown)
3	Cobb	Bovans
4	Marshall	Hyline
5	Hubbard	Dekalb
6	Lohman	Lohman
7	Avian-34	Isa Brown
8	Vencobb	Shaver
9	Hybro	Hisex
10	Indian River	Novogen
11	Cobb-Vantress	Babcock
12	Hy-Line	Amberlink

Table 2.5: Average productive performances of common commercial broiler strains

Sl. No.	Strain	Rearing Period	Body weight	Feed consumption	FCR
1	Ross 308	35 days	2.0-2.2 kg	3.0-3.5 kg	1.70
2	Cobb 400	35 days	2.0-2.3 kg	3.0-3.5 kg	1.72
3	Hubbard	35 days	2.0-2.1 kg	3.0-3.4 kg	1.80

Table 2.6: Average productive performances of common commercial layer strains

Sl. No.	Strain	Total feed consumption/ bird		Age at first egg (days)	Egg production up to 72 weeks (nos.)	Survivability (%)
		Grower (0-19 weeks)	Layer (20-72 weeks)			
1	BV300	6.5-7.0 kg	39-40 kg	130-138	295-320	96
2	BV380	7.5-8.0 kg	43 kg	140-148	285-290	96

3

Breeding of Poultry Judging and Culling in Poultry

Arfan Ali and Ashim Kumar Saikia

Poultry Breeding

Poultry breeding is a scientific practice aimed at enhancing the genetic traits of birds to improve their productivity and quality. Historically, poultry farming began as small-scale backyard operations, but it has now evolved into a major industry. This transformation has been driven by the development of superior breeds for both egg and meat production through advanced breeding and selection techniques. Modern poultry breeds exhibit significantly improved productive capacities, such as higher egg production and better meat quality, compared to their ancestors. Successful poultry breeding requires a deep understanding of the qualities and capabilities of various breeds, allowing breeders to select and combine desirable traits to achieve specific goals, whether for size, weight, egg production, meat quality, or a combination of these factors.

- Poultry production has transitioned from a small-scale backyard venture to a significant industry.
- This growth has been largely driven by the development of superior breeds for egg and meat production, utilizing modern breeding and selection techniques.
- Modern poultry is vastly superior in terms of productive capacity, including the number and size of eggs and the quality and quantity of meat, compared to its ancestors. This progress has been achieved through advancements in both the environment and breeding methods.
- Poultry breeding is a scientific practice aimed at the genetic improvement of birds through successive generations via planned reproduction.
- Successful poultry breeders must have an in-depth understanding of the qualities and capabilities of different poultry breeds to select the right type of birds and combine desirable qualities to a high degree.
- Breeding should be purposeful, and breeders should understand the goal of breeding and the standards to which the birds should be bred, whether

for size, weight, egg production, meat quality, or a combination of these factors.

- The suitability of a male or female bird for breeding purposes is largely determined by the quality of progeny (offspring) they produce.
- For instance, a male bird whose dam (mother) had a high record of egg production, when mated with a female of similar high egg production record, often produces daughters that lay a large number of eggs.

System of Breeding

Breeding systems in poultry can be classified based on whether they aim to increase homozygosity or heterozygosity through random mating, inbreeding, and outbreeding:

A. Random Mating

Random mating is the mating of individuals within a population without any intentional selection based on specific traits or characteristics. It allows for natural genetic variation to be maintained within the population, serving as a baseline for comparing the effects of other breeding methods or environmental factors.

- Random mating involves the mating of individuals without any selection criteria.
- This method is used to establish a control population, which serves as a baseline for comparing and measuring the effects of other breeding systems.
- The control population also helps estimate the influence of environmental factors, thereby enabling a more accurate assessment of true genetic gains achieved through any breeding method.

B. Inbreeding

Inbreeding is defined as the mating between individuals that are more closely related to each other than the average relationship between all individuals in a population.

- It involves mating animals that share one or more common ancestors, leading to an increase in homozygosity.
- For example, inbreeding can include mating a sire with its female offspring or mating closely related individuals.
- Inbreeding can be consistently applied over several generations to fix desired traits but requires careful management to avoid negative consequences such as reduced vigor and increased susceptibility to genetic disorders.

There are three distinct methods of inbreeding:

a) Close inbreeding
b) Strain formation
c) Line breeding

a) Close Inbreeding

- Involves mating between siblings and between parents and progeny.

Examples include full sibling mating and backcrossing progeny to the younger of the parents.

- Sire to daughter
- Son to dam
- Full brother and sister

b) Strain Formation

- Involves developing a small group of animals within a breed or variety with specific desirable characteristics.
- This is a milder form of inbreeding.

Example: The Babcock strain of Single Comb White Leghorn was developed for increased egg weight.

c) Line Breeding

- Involves breeding with an ancestral line and is the most intensive form of backcrossing.
- Typically involves backcrossing to the same parent for several generations in succession.

Examples include half-brother and sister mating or mating animals more distantly related, such as cousins.

Outbreeding

Outbreeding involves mating individuals that are less closely related than the average relationship within the population. It is the opposite of inbreeding and is aimed at introducing genetic diversity.

- Mating between different strains or inbred lines are common forms of outbreeding in poultry breeding.

Methods of Outbreeding (Crossbreeding)

A. **Single or 2-Way Crossing:** Involves crossing individuals from two different strains or lines to combine desirable traits or improve performance.

B. **Three-Way Crossing:** Involves crossing individuals from three different strains or lines to incorporate traits from multiple sources.

C. **Four-Way Crossing:** Involves crossing individuals from four different strains or lines, maximizing genetic diversity and hybrid vigor.

These methods of outbreeding (crossbreeding) are essential strategies in poultry breeding to achieve specific breeding goals such as enhancing productivity, disease resistance, or other desired traits

A. **Single or Two-Way Crossing:** Two different populations (inbred lines, strains, or breeds) are crossed to produce a first filial (F1) generation, which is primarily for commercial purposes rather than breeding.

- The F1 generation typically exhibits hybrid vigor, especially when crossing inbred lines. When two inbred lines of the same breed are crossed, the progeny is referred to as in-crossbred.

A (inbred line) X B (inbred line) = AB (F1 generation)

B. **Three-Way Cross:** In this method, F1 crossbred females (AB) are mated with males of a third line (C) to produce an F2 progeny (ABC).

AB (female) X C (male) = ABC (F2 generation)

C. **Four-Way Cross:** Two different single crosses (AB and CD) are crossed to obtain ABCD.

- A (inbred line) X B (inbred line) = AB
- C (inbred line) X D (inbred line) = CD

AB X CD = ABCD

These methods of crossbreeding are integral in poultry breeding to leverage hybrid vigor and combine desirable traits from different genetic backgrounds effectively.

Crossing for Production of a New Breed

- Developing a breed involves selecting individuals with desired traits, repeatedly breeding them to solidify those traits, and establishing breed standards.
- This process, repeated over generations, leads to a population with consistent traits.
- This process can involve crossbreeding, inbreeding, or other breeding techniques to achieve specific goals, like improved productivity or specific physical characteristics.

  Example: The Cornish breed was developed from crosses involving Aseel, Malay, and English game breeds.

Hybrid Vigor

- Hybrid vigor, also known as heterosis or inbreeding enhancement, refers to the increase in certain characteristics like growth rate, size, fertility, and yield in hybrid organisms compared to their parents.
- This phenomenon occurs because the hybrid offspring inherit enhanced traits due to the genetic contributions from both parents.

Common Egg-Type Hybrid Chicken Strains

- BV-300, BV-380, ISA, Babcock, Bovans, Euribrid, Hyline, HH-260, Dekalb, Keystone, Lohmann, and H & N Nick chick.

Common Meat-Type Hybrid Chicken Strains

- Cobb, Ross, Steggles, Arbor Acres, Hub Chicks, Hybro, Hubbard, Lohmann, Pilch, Starbro, Tegel, Anak-2000, Marshall, Peterson, Samrat-2000, and Avian-34.

These hybrid chicken strains are developed and selected for specific traits such as egg production efficiency or meat yield, contributing significantly to modern poultry production.

Methods of Mating in Poultry

Mating in poultry refers to the pairing of a male and a female for the purpose of reproduction or the production of offspring. Various methods are employed depending on the specific breeding goals and logistical considerations:

a) **Pen Mating**
b) **Stud Mating**
c) **Shift Mating**
d) **Flock mating**
e) **Artifical Insemination**

a) Pen Mating

- **Definition:** Birds are allowed to mate freely within a pen or enclosure containing multiple males and females.
- **Description:** A single male mates with a group of females in a pen during the breeding season.
- **Mating Ratio:** Typically, 1:10-12 females for egg-type birds (e.g., Leghorn) and 1:6-8 for meat-type birds.
- **Pedigreeing:** Possible on both sire's and dam's sides.
- **Labor Requirement:** Moderately higher due to individual pen management.

- **Fertility:** Lower compared to flock mating due to preferential mating.
- **Application:** Commonly used in small-scale or backyard poultry farming where natural mating is preferred.

b) Stud Mating

- **Definition:** Each male bird (stud) is individually paired with a specific female bird.
- **Description:** Males are housed in individual pens (coops), and females are introduced one by one for mating.
- **Frequency:** Ideally, mating occurs twice a week or every 5 days for optimal fertility.
- **Labor Intensity:** High due to individual management hence, less commonly practiced now.
- **Application:** Often used in breeding programs to ensure controlled mating and to track specific genetic crosses.

c) Shift Mating

- **Definition:** Male birds are rotated or shifted between different groups of females to facilitate mating.
- **Description:** Males are rotated among breeding pens to mate with females.

Application

- **Breeding Programs:** It is particularly useful in breeding programs (like family breeding) where multiple males' breeding values need assessment to identify superior individuals.
- **Female Evaluation:** Shift mating allows females to be mated with several males successively, facilitating precise evaluation of their breeding potential.
- **Space Efficiency:** This method enables testing a large number of males in a limited space.
- **Comparison with Pen Mating:** Similar to pen mating, shift mating manages males sequentially across pens. However, it involves relocating males to different pens over time.

Challenges

- **Parentage Accuracy:** A significant challenge is maintaining accurate parentage records. Male fertility persists for 2-3 weeks after removal, complicating pedigree determination.

d) Flock Mating

- **Definition:** All birds within a flock, including both males and females, are allowed to mate freely.
- **Definition:** Flock mating involves keeping a large number of hens with a smaller number of cocks in a ratio typically around 10 hens per cock.

Application

- **Pedigree Records:** Flock mating is preferred in situations where maintaining individual pedigree records is not necessary or feasible.

Advantage

- **Cost Efficiency:** This method reduces operational costs due to a higher number of birds per unit area.

Disadvantages

- **Male Aggression:** Males can become aggressive towards each other, with dominant males preventing others from mating, leading to reduced fertility.
- **Low Fertility:** Dominant males may monopolize mating, resulting in some hens not being adequately fertilized.
- **Pedigree Challenges:** It's difficult to maintain accurate pedigree records due to the communal mating nature, making it less suitable for controlled breeding programs.

e) Artificial Insemination (AI)

- **Definition:** Semen collected from a male bird is manually deposited into the reproductive tract of a female bird.
- **Application:** Widely used in commercial poultry production to control breeding, optimize genetic selection, and prevent the spread of diseases.

These methods of mating are chosen based on factors such as farm size, breeding goals, genetic management strategies, and the need for reproductive efficiency in poultry farming.

Artificial Insemination (AI)

Definition: Artificial Insemination (AI) is a technique where seminal fluid (semen) from a male bird is introduced into the female bird's reproductive tract using a pipette.

Procedure

- **Semen Production:** Typically, a male chicken can produce about 0.5 to 1.0 ml of semen, depending on its body weight. Approximately 0.05 to 0.10 ml of semen is sufficient to inseminate one hen.
- **Timing:** AI is performed during the afternoon when most hens are likely to have laid eggs, ensuring their oviducts are empty.
- **Frequency:** Insemination is usually done twice a week or at least once every five days.

Advantages of AI

- **Efficiency:** One male can fertilize an unlimited number of females without needing extensive breeding equipment.
- **Prevention of Preferential Mating:** AI helps avoid preferential mating, ensuring controlled genetic selection.
- **Accurate Pedigreeing:** Enables precise pedigree records, facilitating genetic improvement programs.
- **Use for Heavy or Old Males:** AI is suitable for heavy or older males that may struggle with natural mating, if the males are too heavy (as in the case of Broad Breasted White Turkey) or too old for natural mating,
- **Cross-Species Hybridization:** Facilitates hybridization between different species, such as chicken-quail hybrids.
- **In Caged Systems:** Essential for obtaining fertile eggs in caged-laying systems.
- **Avoids Trap-Nesting Issues:** Eliminates problems associated with trap-nesting for egg collection.
- **Reduction of Disease Transmission:** Helps reduce or prevent the transmission of sexually transmitted diseases.

Disadvantages of AI

- **Labor Intensive:** Requires more labor compared to natural mating methods.
- **Risk of Contamination:** There is a potential risk of cross-contamination of birds through the insemination equipment, including the spread of infections like paratyphoid.
- **Stress on Birds:** Involves handling of birds during the procedure, which can cause stress, affecting overall welfare.

Selection and Culling

Selection

Selection refers to the process of choosing birds that exhibit desirable characteristics, such as higher meat egg production, superior meat and egg quality, suitability for exhibition, and breeding potential. The success of poultry production heavily relies on the quality of the selected birds and their breed. Selecting subpar males and hens for the breeding flock can lead to significant financial losses, even with optimal feed, management, and disease control practices in place.

Therefore, selection should be guided by the specific production goals, whether for eggs, meat, or a combination of both. To establish a strong foundation stock, consider the following key points:

1. **Desired Characteristics:** Clearly define the traits you aim to enhance, such as egg production, growth rate, feed efficiency, or disease resistance.
2. **Breed Suitability:** Choose breeds known for excelling in the desired characteristics. For instance, Leghorns are renowned for egg production, while Cornish are preferred for meat production.
3. **Performance Records:** Utilize records and data on individual bird performance to make informed selection decisions.
4. **Health and Vitality:** Select birds that show robust health, vigor, and resistance to diseases.
5. **Conformation and Structure:** Ensure birds have the appropriate body structure and conformation for their intended purpose.
6. **Genetic Diversity:** Maintain genetic diversity within the flock to prevent inbreeding and promote long-term health and productivity.
7. **Environmental Adaptability:** Choose birds that are well-suited to the local climate and environmental conditions.

By focusing on these fundamental aspects, poultry breeders can enhance the quality and productivity of their flocks, ensuring a profitable and sustainable poultry operation.

Selection for Egg Production

When selecting birds for egg production, it is crucial to determine whether the focus is on the number, size, or color of the eggs. The selection process should prioritize breeds that exhibit all the characteristics of excellent layers, including:

- **Quick Maturity:** Birds that reach reproductive age rapidly and begin laying eggs sooner.
- **Good Stamina:** Birds that can sustain high egg production over a long period.
- **Alertness:** Birds that are active and responsive, indicating good health and vitality.
- **Good Conformation:** Birds with the appropriate body structure that supports efficient egg production.
- **Capacity to Lay a Large Number of Standard Size Eggs:** Birds that consistently produce eggs of uniform size and quality

Some of the breeds and hybrid strains that are highly recommended for their prolific egg production capabilities include:

- **White Leghorns:** Known for their exceptional laying ability and adaptability
- **Hybrid Strains:** BV-300, BV-380 Babcock, Ranishavers, Unichix, Hyline, Hisex, HH-260, and Poone Pearls are among the top choices for producing a large number of good-sized eggs. These hybrids have been selectively bred to maximize egg production efficiency and quality.

By carefully selecting birds with these desirable traits, poultry producers can ensure a high level of egg production that meets their specific requirements.

Body Conformation for Higher Egg Production

To ensure a bird can lay a large number of eggs, it should possess a body with the following characteristics:

- **Flat Broad Back:** The back should be flat and broad, providing adequate space for internal organs.
- **Good Depth of Body:** The depth of the body should increase towards the abdomen, especially in laying condition, indicating ample space for egg production.
- **Good Span Between Pubic Bones and Keel Bone**: This space should be wide, indicating a bird's ability to lay large eggs consistently.
- **Thin, Straight Pubic Bones Set Well Apart:** Ensures less resistance during egg laying.
- **Good Quality of Skin:** The skin should be loose, pliable, and velvety, indicating overall good health and vitality.
- **Legs Set Well Apart and Short:** Legs should be well-spaced and short, with smooth and clean shanks, and short nails to ensure stability and support.

- **Reasonably Long Keel Bone:** A longer keel bone provides more support and indicates a bird with good skeletal structure.
- **Well-Proportioned:** The bird should be well-proportioned with skeletal development consistent with its size, ensuring a balanced body capable of sustaining high egg production.

These physical traits contribute to the overall health, stamina, and egg-laying capacity of the bird, making them essential considerations for selection in egg production.

Selection for Meat Production

For meat production, the selected birds should ideally weigh around 2 kg at 10-12 weeks of age, although high-quality broilers can achieve this weight much earlier, in about 5-6 weeks. A small, compact bird of this weight is preferred over a heavier one because it is cost-effective and provides just enough meat for one meal, thus minimizing wastage.

Key Characteristics for Meat Birds

- **Rapid Growth:** Birds that can quickly attain the desired weight.
- **Compact Size:** A small, compact bird that meets the weight requirement without excess bulk.
- **Fleshy and Heavy:** Birds that are very fleshy and have a substantial amount of meat.

Table 3.1: Breeds and Hybrid Strains for Meat Production

Sl. No.	Meat type breeds	Hybrid Meat Strains
1	Plymouth Rocks	Indian River
2	Cornish	Venkob
3	New Hampshire	Ross Broilers
4	Sussex	Hubchix
5	Orpington	Unichix
6	Wyandotte	Arbor Acres
7	Jersey Giant	Cobb
8	Brahma	Hubbard
9	Delaware	Marshall
10	Dorking	Avian-34
11	Buckeye	Anak-2000
12	Australorp	Tegel
13	Rhode Island Red	
14	Cochin	

These breeds and hybrid strains are recognized for their rapid growth, fleshy build, and suitability for meat production.

Culling

Culling is the process of removing birds from a flock that do not meet the desired standards for which they were bred, whether for egg production or meat purposes. It involves eliminating uneconomical and non-productive birds, ensuring that only the best individuals contribute to the flock's productivity and genetic improvement. Both culling and selection are the two sides of a coin.

Distinction from Selection

While culling focuses on removing inferior birds, selection involves choosing the best individuals from a flock for breeding purposes. Selection aims to enhance desirable traits and improve overall flock quality over successive generations.

Importance

Culling plays a crucial role in maintaining the efficiency of the flock:

- **Resource Efficiency:** Uneconomical birds consume the same resources as productive ones, increasing maintenance costs. Removing non-performers optimizes resource allocation.
- **Continual Process:** Culling should be an ongoing practice throughout the year, applicable to both small and large poultry farms. It ensures that the flock remains productive and healthy.
- **Uniformity and Disease Prevention:** Periodic culling of growing stock helps maintain flock uniformity and prevents the spread of diseases within the flock.

Indicators of Sickness and Lack of Vigor

Recognizing signs of illness or reduced vigor is essential for effective culling:

- Young chickens appearing dull or lethargic.
- Birds huddling in corners instead of actively feeding or moving.
- Droopy feathers or plumage lacking its normal luster.
- Chickens exhibiting grey or pearly eyes, indicating potential health issues.

Methods of Culling

Effective culling methods include

- **Non-Performers:** Birds failing to meet production standards should be removed promptly to maintain overall flock productivity.
- **Health Issues:** Birds with chronic health problems or signs of disease should be isolated and culled to prevent spread within the flock.
- **Physical Defects:** Birds with physical abnormalities that impair productivity or breeding potential should be culled to maintain flock health.
- **Ageing Birds:** Older birds passed their prime production age should be culled to make room for younger, more productive birds.
- **Behavioral Problems:** Birds displaying aggressive behavior that disrupts flock harmony should be considered for culling to maintain a stress-free environment.

Regular and systematic culling ensures that only the best-performing and healthiest birds contribute to the flock's success. By combining careful selection and diligent culling practices, poultry breeders can achieve and maintain a high-quality flock that consistently meets their production goals.

Culling of Growers

Culling growers is a critical practice in poultry farming to maintain flock quality and productivity. Here are key considerations for culling growers:

1. **Poor Feathering:** Some birds may exhibit poor feathering up to six or eight weeks of age. This condition can be due to overcrowding, dietary deficiencies, or inherited traits. Birds with persistent poor feathering should not be used for breeding purposes. Instead, they should be identified, marked, and sold as table birds at around 10 to 12 weeks of age.
2. **Body Shape and Fleshing Capacity:** Birds with poor body shape and inadequate fleshing capacity should be culled. These characteristics include:
    - Long-legged birds that lack compactness.
    - Narrow-bodied birds that do not meet breed standards.
    - Birds with crooked breast bones, which affect their growth and health.
    - Those with defective tail carriage, which may indicate underlying health or genetic issues.

Culling ensures that only birds with optimal growth potential, physical conformation, and health are retained in the flock. This practice helps in maintaining uniformity, preventing the spread of undesirable traits, and ultimately enhancing overall flock performance and profitability in poultry production.

Culling of Layers

Culling layers is crucial for maintaining the profitability and efficiency of a laying flock. Here are important considerations for culling layers:

1. **Profitability and Egg Production:** The profitability of a laying flock is closely tied to egg production. Since feed costs constitute a significant portion of the total expenses (approximately 60%), it is economically prudent to cull poor layers promptly.
2. **Identification of Poor Layers:** Birds that consistently produce below-average egg yields should be identified and culled from the flock. This includes birds that show a decline in egg production over time or those that fail to reach expected production levels for their breed.
3. **Culling Criteria:**
    - **Consistent Low Production:** Birds that consistently lay fewer eggs than their peers.
    - **Early Decline in Production:** Birds that have initially performed well but have shown a sudden or prolonged decline in egg production.
    - **Health Issues:** Birds with chronic health problems affecting their ability to lay eggs.
4. **Optimizing Flock Performance:** Regular and systematic culling helps maintain high productivity levels within the flock. It prevents the wastage of feed resources on non-productive birds and allows for the replacement of poor performers with younger, more productive layers.

By implementing effective culling practices, poultry farmers can ensure that their laying flocks remain efficient, profitable, and capable of meeting production targets consistently. This approach contributes to overall farm sustainability and profitability in egg production.

Judging and Culling of Poultry

Judging of poultry involves physical examination of a bird to assess quality and suitability for different purposes viz. meat production, egg production or exhibition. It is a careful observation, handling and assessment of the physical characteristics of the bird with predetermined goal.

Objectives

The process of judging and culling poultry serves several important objectives in poultry farming:

1. **Identifying Breed Type:** To recognize specimens that closely adheres to the ideal characteristics of their breed type.
2. **Selecting Breeders:** To choose superior birds as breeding stock for future generations, ensuring genetic progress in desired traits.
3. **Culling Unproductive Birds:** To remove birds from the flock that do not meet production expectations, thereby optimizing overall productivity.
4. **Cost Reduction:** To minimize the cost of rearing by timely culling of non-performing birds, which reduces feed and maintenance expenses.

Procedure

A. Physical Characteristics Method

- **Judging Basis:** Evaluation is based on the overall appearance and specific body characteristics of birds according to their breed standards.
- **Timing:** Judging typically occurs after birds reach sexual maturity, around 26 to 28 weeks of age for chickens.
- **Performance Categories:** Birds are categorized as good layers, poor layers, or non-layers (those that have not started laying eggs).

This method ensures that only the most suitable birds are retained for breeding and production purposes, contributing to the efficiency and profitability of the poultry operation.

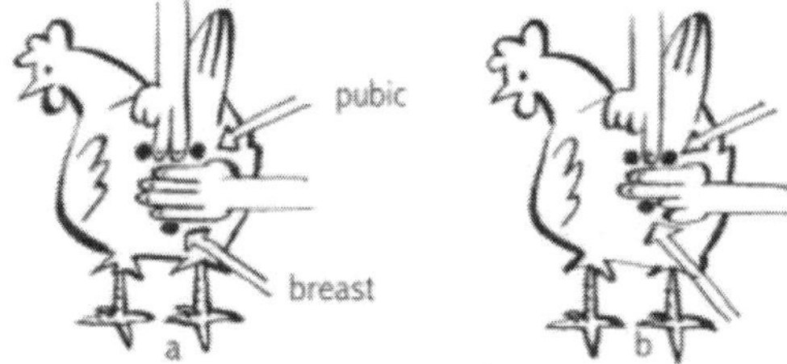

Fig: 3.1

Table 3.2: Characteristics to be observed for judging of layer birds

Parameters	Good layer	Poor layer	Non-layer
Plumage	Initially bright, dulls over time	Brighter	Always bright
Comb and Wattles	Large, red, indicating health	Small, less warm, shrunken, indicating poor health	Underdeveloped, indicating immaturity
Eyes	Big, active, bright, indicating alertness	Small, dull, indicating lethargy	Small, dull, indicating lethargy

Vent	Oblong, moist, pink, indicating health	Less oblong, moist/ dry, pink, indicating dehydration or stress	Round, dry, yellow, indicating poor health
Distance between two pubic bones	At least 3 fingers width, indicating good egg-laying potential	Less than 3 fingers width, indicating reduced egg-laying potential	Maximum 1 finger width, indicating immaturity or non-laying status
Distance between tip of breast bone and pubic bones	At least 4 fingers width, soft, pliable, indicating good body condition	Less than 4 fingers width, not very soft, indicating poorer body condition	Rubbery, very hard, maximum 2 fingers width, indicating very poor body condition

Explanation

- **Plumage:** Initially bright feathers that dull over time may indicate a normal shedding cycle. Constantly bright plumage suggests good health and grooming habits.
- **Comb and Wattles:** A large, red comb and wattles are signs of good blood circulation and overall health. Small, shrunken ones indicate potential health issues or stress.
- **Eyes:** Large, bright, and active eyes indicate alertness and vitality. Small and dull eyes may suggest lethargy or illness.
- **Vent:** An oblong, moist, and pink vent indicates good reproductive health. Changes such as dryness or yellow coloration may signal dehydration, stress, or illness.
- **Distance between two pubic bones:** A wider gap (at least 3 fingers width) between pubic bones suggests good egg-laying potential and pelvic width. Narrower gaps indicate reduced potential or immaturity.
- **Distance between breast bone and pubic bones:** A wider gap (at least 4 fingers width), with soft and pliable tissues, indicates good body condition and potential for sustained egg production. Narrower gaps with firmer or rubbery tissues suggest poor body condition and reduced egg-laying capacity.

Definitions

- **Pliable:** Soft, flexible, and yielding to touch, indicating good muscle tone and health.
- **Rubbery:** Tough, rigid, and unyielding to touch, indicating poor muscle tone and health, often associated with reduced productivity.

Table 3.3: Distinguished features for judging good and poor performers

Parameters	Good birds	Poor birds
Head	Strongly feminine in females and masculine in males; well proportioned, square and broad at the top,	Masculine in females (crow or eagle-headed); narrow and tapering at the end
Comb and Wattles	Full, red, waxy and velvety	Dry, scaly, shrivelled, cold, coarse.
Beak	Stocky, well-curved.	Long, thin, sharp-pointed.
Eyes	Full, bright, alert.	Dull, sleepy
Neck	Short, stocky.	Long, thin.
Body	Capacious.	Not so capacious.
Back	Broad, straight.	Narrow, pinched, crooked.
Side	Deep, straight	Shallow, barrel shaped
Keel bone	Long, curved	Short, crooked
Pubic bone	Wide apart, thin, pliable	Thick, stiff, close together
Skin	Thin, soft, oily	Thick, dry, rough
Abdomen	Large, soft, free from lumps of fat	Small, hard, full of fat
Vent	Full, large, moist	Small, dry
Feather	Compact	Loose
Shank	Thin, soft in back	Thick, rounded in back
Toe nails	Stocky, well-curved	Long, thin, sharp-pointed
Temperament	Friendly, happy	Shy, nervous, squakes
Crop fill	Full	Not full
Pigmentation	Bleaching occurs with laying age	Non-bleaching of body parts

A. Score card method

Table 3.4: Score card for judging male birds

Particulars	Maximum scores	Score obtained			
		Bird 1	Bird 2	Bird 3	Bird 4
Head	20				
Neck	5				
Body	40				
Legs	10				
Temperament	20				
Appetite	5				
Total score	100				

Table 3.5: Score card for judging female birds

Particulars	Maximum scores	Score obtained			
		Bird 1	Bird 2	Bird 3	Bird 4
Head	10				
Neck	5				
Body	50				
Legs	10				
Temperament	10				
Appetite	5				
Pigmentation	10				
Total score	100				

B. Depigmentation as a tool for judging layer birds

Depigmentation, or bleaching, serves as a valuable indicator for assessing the persistency of egg production in layer birds. Xanthophylls, a pigment derived primarily from feed sources such as yellow maize, is stored in various body parts of the bird. As the bird ages and progresses through its laying cycle, it gradually loses this pigment.

During the latter stages of egg production, typically in the last 20 weeks when egg production decreases, the pigments reappear in reverse order. This phenomenon provides insights into the bird's reproductive cycle and can help in assessing the health and productivity of laying hens.

Table 3.6: Order of de-pigmentation in layer birds

Tissue bleached	No. of eggs
Vent	When first egg is laid
Eye lids	6-8
Ear lobes	9-10
Beaks	11-35
Underside of feet	66
Front of shanks	95
Back of shanks	159
Top of toes	170
Hock joint	180

4

Indian Native Poultry Breeds and Their Importance in Rural India

Mustafizur Rahman and Rafiqul Islam

India's indigenous poultry breeds play a crucial role in rural livelihoods, providing a sustainable source of nutrition and income. These native breeds are well-adapted to the local environmental conditions, demonstrating remarkable resilience and disease resistance. Despite their lower production potential compared to commercial breeds, their economic value and cultural significance make them indispensable in the rural context.

Indigenous Fowls of India

- India has a population of 217.80 million indigenous (Desi) chickens, representing 25.57% of the total poultry population (851.81 million) in India (BAHS, 2023, GOI).
- A total of 20 indigenous chicken breeds, 3 duck breeds, and 1 geese breed have been registered under the ICAR-National Bureau of Animal Genetics Resources (NBAGR) to date (Table 4.1 & 4.2).
- Indigenous fowls are typically reared under a backyard system, often referred to as "backyard poultry," with minimal focus on housing and feeding.
- Despite their lower production potential, these breeds are well-adapted to local environmental conditions. They are hardy and resistant to most common avian diseases.
- The prices of eggs and meat from local chickens are 100 to 150 times higher than those of their commercial counterparts.
- Indigenous chickens are also known as "village poultry," "family poultry," or "scavenging poultry" in many parts of the world.

Indigenous Chicken Breeds in India

India is home to 20 registered indigenous chicken breeds, each with unique characteristics and regional adaptations. These breeds are an important part of the country's agricultural biodiversity. The following is a detailed description of these breeds:

Table 4.1: Indian native chicken breeds

Sl. No.	Breed	Region	Characteristics	Body Weight (kg)	Age at Sexual Maturity (days)	Annual Egg Production	Egg Weight (g)	Egg Colour
1	Ankleshwar	Ankleshwar, Bharuch, Narmada (Gujarat)	White to light grey, brown, golden plumage; red comb (single/rose type)	Male: 1.76, Female: 1.49	181 days	81	34.3	Cream
2	Aseel	Coastal Andhra Pradesh, Dantewada (CG)	Tall, pugnacious, high stamina, fighting qualities	Cock: 3-4, Hen: 2-3	196 days	92	50	Light Brown
3	Bursa	Maharashtra, Gujarat	White plumage with black neck, back, tail, reddish-brown shoulders and wings	Cock: 0.85-1.25, Hen: 0.80-1.20	5-7 months	40-55	28-38	Light Brown
4	Chittagong	Meghalaya, Tripura, Bangladesh	Large, strong, hardy, quarrelsome; white with gold wing markings	Cock: 3.5-4.5, Hen: 3.0-4.0	217 days	130	52	Brown
5	Danki	Andhra Pradesh, Odisha	Attractive, red glossy plumage, darker neck, no wattle	Cock: 3.12, Hen: 2.22	6-8 months	25-35	46	Brown
6	Daothigir	Kokrajhar, Chirang, Udalguri, Baksa (Assam)	Yellowish brown/red males; barred black and white females; large red comb	Cock: 1.79, Hen: 1.63	6-8 months	60-70	44.42	Brown
7	Ghagus	Karnataka, Andhra Pradesh	Brown/black plumage, golden neck feathers	Cock: 2.16, Hen: 1.43	5-7 months	45-60	45	Light Brown
8	Harringhata Black	West Bengal	Small black bird, red comb and wattles, white shanks	Cock: 1.5, Hen: 1.2	78	130	45	Light Brown
9	Kadaknath	Western Madhya Pradesh, Rajasthan, Gujarat	Bluish black plumage, slate-like skin, beak, shanks, toes, soles, black organs	Cock: 1.5, Hen: 1.0	185 days	80	46.8	Light Brown

10	Kalasthi	Andhra Pradesh	Bluish black/brown plumage; cocks with golden neck and wings	Cock: 2.48, Hen: 1.85	6-8 months	30-40	42.91	-
11	Kashmir Favorella	Kashmir	Small, feathered comb, thrives at high altitude	Cock: 1.72, Hen: 1.25	210 days	60-85	50	Light Brown
12	Miri	Sivasagar, Dhemaji, Lakhimpur (Assam)	Black/brown/white plumage, white/yellow shanks, red earlobes	Cock: 1.2-1.3, Hen: 0.90-1.0	168 days	60-70	29-42	Light Brown
13	Nicobari	Nicobar Islands	Black, brown, white strains; small, round, compact body	Male: 1.2, Hen: 1.0	177-200 days	140-150	48	Brown
14	Punjab Brown	Punjab, Haryana	Meat type, brown plumage, black spots/stripes on males	Cock: 3.0-4.0, Hen: 2.0-2.5	150-180 days	60-80	45	Brown
15	Tellicherry	Kerala, Puducherry	Small, round, black plumage with bluish tinge	Cock: 1.62, Hen: 1.24	5-8 months	60-80	48	Tinted
16	Mewari	Mewar (Rajasthan)	Small to medium, yellow shank and skin, mostly brown plumage	Cock: 1.90, Hen: 1.24	142 days	37-52	35	Cream
17	Kaunayen	Manipur	Elongated body, long neck and legs, black/brown plumage	Cock: 3.01, Hen: 2.32	5-7 months	35	47	Brown
18	Hansli	Odisha	Similar to Aseel, used for cock fighting, red comb, wattle, face, earlobe	Cock: 2.5-3.0, Hen: 1.5-2.0	6 months	50-60	50	Brown
19	Uttara	Uttarakhand	Feathered shank, resistant to cold, white skin, yellow shank	Cock: 1.3, Hen: 1.1	6 months	125-160	50	Light Brown
20	Aravali	Gujarat	Heat tolerant, birchen plumage in males, shaft/laced in females	Cock: 1.99, Hen: 1.62	6 months	72	45	Brown

Indigenous duck breed

Indigenous ducks in India are believed to be descendants of the Mallard and are primarily bred for their eggs and meat. Among the various indigenous duck breeds in India, only three duck breeds are registered under ICAR-NBAGR, Karnal. They are *Pati*, *Maithili* and *Andamani* ducks.

Table 4.2: Indian native duck breeds/varieties

Sl. No.	Breed	Region	Characteristics	Body Weight (kg)	Age at Sexual Maturity	Annual Egg Production	Egg Weight (g)	Egg Colour
1	Pati	Assam	Dark brown plumage with greenish black head; black and white tail feathers	Male: 1.9, Female: 1.8	160-190 days	75-93	60	Creamy white
2	Maithili	Bihar	Uniform light/dark brown feathers; dark brown to ash-colored plumage in drakes	Male: 1.45, Female: 1.37	159-223 days	33-71	50	Creamy white or bluish white
3	Andamani	Andaman	Black plumage with white marking under neck extending to belly	Male: 1.41, Female: 1.27	159-223 days	266	60	Creamy white
4	Kuttanad	Kerala	Chara: Greenish black head plumage; Chemballi: Dull greenish black head plumage	-	129 days	200	70	white
5	Arni	Tamil Nadu	Sanyasi: Saffron plumage with or without white ring; Keeri: Black and brown mix	Male: 1.8, Female: 1.4	182-189 days	160-200	60-64	Creamy white or bluish white
6	Nageswari	Assam (originally Sylhet, BD)	Drake: Dull brownish black head; duck: Blackish brown with white neck plumage	Male: 1.42, Female: 1.26	180-195 days	100-120	60	Bluish tinge
7	Kuzi	Odisha	Males have black, mottled brown plumage colour with dark green heads, while females have mottled brown heads and reddish brown breasts. Body weight: 1.7 to 1.8 kg; Age at sexual maturity: 6-8 months; Egg weight: 70 g ; Egg colour: White or Creamy white	1.032-1.120	-	218	-	-

Indigenous geese breed

Kashmir Anz

- **Origin and Recognition:** Kashmir Anz is the first and currently the only recognized domestic geese breed in India.
- **Physical Characteristics:** These geese exhibit varying colors including cinnamon, white, and combinations of cinnamon and white. Their beak color ranges from black to yellow.
- **Varieties:** The breed includes two distinct strains or types known as 'Safed Anz' and 'Katchur Anz'.
- **Body Weight:** Adult ganders (males) typically weigh around 3.82 kg, while adult geese (females) weigh about 3.34 kg on average.
- **Egg Production:** Each Kashmir Anz goose lays approximately 12 eggs per year. These eggs have white shells and weigh around 137 grams on average.

This breed is valued for its distinct appearance and moderate egg production, making it significant in domestic geese farming in Kashmir and potentially other regions.

Role of Indigenous Chicken in Rural Ecosystem of India

1. **Nutritional Security:** Indigenous chicken provides a low-cost source of animal protein through eggs and meat, contributing significantly to combatting malnutrition in rural communities.
2. **Livelihood Support:** It plays a crucial role in the income generation and livelihoods of rural families, thereby fostering the overall development of the poultry sector.
3. **Waste Conversion:** Backyard poultry efficiently converts kitchen wastes, vegetable scraps, green grass, and fallen grains into high-quality animal protein in the form of eggs and meat, reducing waste and enhancing sustainability.
4. **Employment Generation:** Indigenous chicken rearing offers employment opportunities, particularly for unemployed rural youth and women who may have limited access to other income-generating activities.
5. **Utilization of Family Labor:** It optimizes family labor resources by engaging children, elderly members, and others who may not participate in other agricultural activities, thereby improving rural family incomes.

6. **Contribution to Livelihood Indicators:** Indigenous chicken farming positively impacts income levels, nutrition, food security, savings, and promotes gender equality among rural populations.
7. **Empowerment of Women:** Given that women are often involved in indigenous chicken rearing, it enhances their decision-making abilities and involvement in family affairs, leading to empowerment within rural communities.
8. **Cultural and Social Significance:** Indigenous chickens hold cultural and religious importance, being used in rituals to appease gods, spirits, and for traditional ceremonies marking agricultural activities, weddings, births, and deaths.
9. **Manure Production:** Approximately, 15 local chickens can produce 1–1.2 kg of manure daily, which serves as valuable fertilizer for vegetable gardens, fruit trees, and other crops within the village, promoting sustainable agricultural practices.

Indigenous chicken farming not only addresses nutritional and economic needs but also preserves cultural heritage and promotes sustainable practices within rural ecosystems in India.

Constraints of Indigenous Chicken Farming

1. **Disease Outbreaks:** Indigenous chickens are susceptible to diseases such as Ranikhet disease (Newcastle disease), Gumboro disease, Salmonellosis, and Coccidiosis due to inadequate preventive measures. These diseases can cause high mortality rates, sometimes up to 100%, among indigenous flocks.
2. **High Chick Mortality:** A significant challenge in indigenous chicken farming is high chick mortality, with up to 60% of chicks dying in their early life stages, especially during winter due to improper brooding management and exposure to chilling conditions.
3. **Predation:** Indigenous chickens reared under free-range systems are vulnerable to predation, leading to losses, particularly among young and weaker birds. Predators often target these birds, impacting the overall flock size and productivity.
4. **Lower Production Potential:** Compared to commercial breeds, indigenous chickens have lower production potential in terms of egg and meat production due to their inferiro genetic makeup. They expend considerable energy in scavenging and evading predators in free-range systems, resulting in suboptimal production performance.

5. **Lack of Scientific Knowledge:** Many indigenous chicken farmers, predominantly women and children, lack scientific knowledge of optimal poultry management practices. This includes deficiencies in understanding housing, feeding, brooding, medication, and vaccination protocols, which contribute to high mortality rates and poor overall performance.
6. **Limited Access to Inputs and Services:** Access to quality inputs such as vaccines, medications, and improved breeds is often limited for indigenous chicken farmers, hindering their ability to improve productivity and mitigate disease risks effectively.
7. **Market Access and Price Fluctuations:** Indigenous chicken farmers often face challenges in accessing markets with fair prices for their produce. Market fluctuations and inconsistent demand can affect their income stability and profitability.

Addressing these constraints requires targeted interventions such as capacity building in poultry management practices, improved access to veterinary services and inputs, and enhancing market linkages for indigenous chicken farmers. These efforts can contribute to sustainable and resilient indigenous poultry farming systems in rural areas.

5

Improved Backyard Poultry and Their Importance in Rural Eco-System

Rafiqul Islam and Mustafizur Rahman

Desi chickens reared under backyard systems face several constraints such as lower productivity, higher incidence of disease outbreaks, high mortality rates during the early stages of life, and predation. Despite these challenges, the demand for rural backyard poultry is high, particularly among tribal households in rural areas. Small rural producers typically rear colored birds and produce brown-shelled eggs from Desi backyard poultry, catering to the requirements of rural consumers.

To address these issues, there is a need for specific rural poultry production programs. The Indian Council of Agricultural Research (ICAR), New Delhi, initiated a project to upgrade indigenous low input technology birds through the All India Coordinated Research Project on Poultry (AICRPP) in various parts of the country. This initiative aims to evolve improved rural backyard poultry breeds.

Special Features of Improved Rural Backyard or Low Input Technology (LIT) Poultry

- **Enhanced Egg Production:** These birds produce between 125-150 eggs per annum, significantly higher than the Desi hens.
- **Increased Body Weight:** They attain a body weight of 1.1-1.5 kg at 8 weeks of age, which is higher than Desi chickens.
- **Attractive Color Patterns:** The germplasm exhibits more attractive color patterns than Desi hens. The colored plumage provides camouflaging abilities to protect against predators.
- **Adaptability:** These birds can adapt well to harsh environmental conditions, including poor housing, management, and feeding.
- **Absence of Broodiness:** The absence of broodiness results in higher egg production.

- **Nutritional Value:** The eggs and meat have similar nutritional value, aroma, and taste as Desi hens.
- **Lower Fat Content:** The meat has less fat content, making it suitable for consumption by elderly people.
- **Resilience:** These birds thrive and perform better even in adverse environmental conditions.
- **Disease Resistance:** They are sturdy and resistant to most common poultry diseases due to high immune competence.
- **Feed Efficiency:** These birds perform well on diets high in crude fiber and have better feed efficiency with low energy and protein diets based on common rural feed ingredients like rice bran, broken rice, and small millets (foxtail millet, finger millet, pearl millet, etc.).
- **Low Mortality Rate:** Mortality is less than 2% up to eight weeks of age.
- **Heavier Eggs:** The eggs are heavier (55 to 63 g), with brown or tinted shells that are attractive and resemble Desi hen eggs.
- **High Fertility and Hatchability:** Fertility and hatchability rates are 87% and 80%, respectively, allowing farmers to get more chicks compared to Desi hens by using broody hens.
- **Natural Foraging:** These birds perform well in backyard conditions, foraging on green grass and insects available in the fields.
- **Improved Crossbreeding:** The performance of Desi hens can also be enhanced by crossing them with males developed for backyard farming.

Improved backyard poultry breeds offer significant benefits for rural ecosystems by providing a sustainable source of animal protein, enhancing rural livelihoods, and contributing to the overall development of the poultry sector.

Table 5.1: Varieties Developed for Rural Backyard Poultry in India

Variety	Developed By	Adult Body Weight (kg)	Age at Sexual Maturity (days)	Annual Egg Production (numbers)	Egg Weight (g)
Giriraja	KVAFSU, Bangalore	Male: 2.0-2.5	155-160	130-150	52-55
Vanaraja	ICAR-Directorate on Poultry Research, Hyderabad	Male: 2.4-2.8	175-180	110	-
Gramapriya	ICAR-DRP, Hyderabad	Male: 1.8-2.0	170-175	160-180	-
Kamrupa	Assam Agricultural University, Guwahati	Male: 1.7-1.8	150-170	140-150	-
Srinidhi	ICAR-DRP, Hyderabad	Male: 1.7-2.0	165-170	140-150	-
Kuroiler	Kegg Farms, Gurgaon, New Delhi	Male: 2.0 (at 8 weeks)	180	160-180	-
Rainbow Rooster	Indbro Research & Breeding Farms, Hyderabad	Male: 2.5-3.5 (at 20 weeks)	180	150	-
Jharsim	BAU, Ranchi	Male: 1.6-1.8	175-180	175-180	-
Gramalaxmi	BAU, Ranchi	Male: 1.6-1.8	175-180	175-180	-
CARI Debendra	ICAR-CARI	Male: 1.1-1.2 (at 8 weeks)	155-160	190-200	-
CARI Nirbheek	ICAR-CARI	Male: 1.35 (at 20 weeks)	176	198	54
CARI Upcari	ICAR-CARI	Male: 1.285 (at 20 weeks)	165	222	60
CARI Hitcari	ICAR-CARI	Male: 1.320 (at 20 weeks)	178	200	61
CARI Shyama	ICAR-CARI	Male: 1.120 (at 20 weeks)	170	210	53

Notes on Specific Varieties

1. CARI Shyama

- Cross between Indian native chicken Kadaknath and CARI-red.
- Most internal organs (muscles and tissues) show characteristic black pigmentation.

2. CARI Hitcari

- Cross between Indian native chicken with naked neck plumage and CARI-red.
- Well adapted to tropical climate, especially hot and humid coastal regions.

3. CARI Upcari

- An egg-type improved backyard chicken.
- Cross between Indian native chicken with frizzle plumage and CARI-red.
- Well adapted to tropical climates, particularly in arid zones.

4. CARI Nirbheek

- An egg-type backyard chicken.
- Product of a cross between Indian native breed Aseel and CARI-red.

These improved varieties of backyard poultry offer enhanced productivity, resilience, and adaptability, making them suitable for the rural ecosystem and contributing to the overall well-being of rural communities.

Role of Improved Backyard Chicken in Rural India

Backyard poultry farming is a time-honored tradition in rural India, blending seamlessly into the livestock rearing practices of local communities. This method, characterized by its low-tech approach and minimal capital investment, plays a significant role in enhancing rural livelihoods. Here's a detailed look at the contributions and benefits of improved backyard chicken farming:

1. Traditional and Eco-Friendly Farming

- Backyard poultry farming is deeply rooted in rural traditions, offering an organic approach to poultry keeping with no harmful residues in eggs and meat. This method supports eco-friendly farming practices and contributes to sustainable agriculture.

2. Pest Control and Manure Production

- These birds are actively engaged in pest control, reducing the need for chemical pesticides. Additionally, they provide valuable manure, enhancing soil fertility and contributing to organic farming practices.

3. Cultural and Ceremonial Significance

- Improved backyard poultry is integral to various festivals and traditional ceremonies in rural areas, reflecting its cultural importance and role in community life.

4. Economic and Nutritional Benefits

- Backyard poultry offers a supplementary income source with minimal investment. The system ensures the availability of eggs and meat even in remote areas, improving food security and nutrition.

5. Adaptability and Low Maintenance

- Local breeds used in backyard poultry are well-adapted to the local environment, providing resilience against predators and diseases. This adaptability makes them a viable option for rural poor communities.

6. Scavenging System

- In the scavenging system practiced in tropical countries like India and Bangladesh, birds are allowed to roam in a fenced area where they forage for food. They are not confined like in commercial systems but are provided with night shelters. This system reduces feed costs as the birds scavenge for a significant portion of their diet, supplemented by a small amount of grains.

7. Enhanced Production and Care

- Compared to free-range systems, improved backyard poultry systems offer better growth rates and egg production. This is achieved through supplementary feeding, proper housing, and enhanced care. Uniformity in flock management also contributes to improved productivity.

8. Efficient Use of Resources

- Farmers efficiently utilize waste grains, household scraps, and leftover kitchen waste for feeding the birds, promoting sustainability and reducing waste.

9. Requirements for Increased Returns

To maximize returns from backyard poultry, certain measures are necessary:

- **High-Yielding Breeds:** Selecting birds with good scavenging ability and high production potential.
- **Supplementary Feeding and Housing:** Providing additional feed and proper housing to boost production.
- **Vaccination and Medication:** Implementing a regular vaccination and medication schedule to minimize disease-related mortality.

Improved backyard chicken farming in rural India enhances livelihoods by offering economic benefits, cultural significance, and nutritional value while supporting sustainable farming practices.

6

Different Rearing System of Poultry and Their Merits and Demerits

Mihir Sarma and Arfan Ali

Poultry rearing systems vary in scale and complexity, each suited to different production needs and environments. This chapter explores the main poultry housing systems, detailing their advantages and disadvantages to help in selecting the most appropriate method for various farming scenarios.

Housing Systems of Poultry

Generally, there are four types of housing systems in poultry, they are

1. Free range or extensive system,
2. Semi-intensive system,
3. Folding unit system and
4. Intensive system.

1. Free Range or Extensive System

Description: The free-range system is one of the oldest **methods of poultry r**earing. It involves allowing poultry to roam freely over a designated area during the day while providing shelter only for the night.

Feeding

- **Primary Source:** Foraging is the main source of nutrition for the birds. They feed on available natural resources such as insects, plants, and grains found in their environment.
- **Supplementary Feeding:** Minimal supplementary feeding may be provided, often in the form of a handful of grains each morning and evening.

Housing

- **Day time:** Birds are allowed to roam freely during the day, which helps them find a significant amount of their food through foraging.
- **Night time:** Shelter is provided for the birds at night to protect them from predators and adverse weather conditions.

Capacity

- **Scale:** Typically involves a very small number of birds, often ranging from 10 to 12 birds per farmer's family.

Advantages

- **Low Cost:** Minimal investment in infrastructure and feed as birds primarily forage for their food.
- **Natural Behavior:** Allows birds to exhibit natural behaviors, which can contribute to their well-being.

Disadvantages

- **Limited Production:** Not suitable for commercial poultry production due to the limited number of birds and the reliance on foraging.
- **Predation Risks:** Birds are more exposed to predators and environmental hazards, which can impact their survival and health.

Profitability: While rearing birds in this system can be profitable on a small scale due to low feed costs, it is generally not viable for large-scale commercial poultry operations.

2. Semi-Intensive System

Description: The semi-intensive system is a hybrid approach to poultry rearing that combines elements of both free range and intensive systems. It includes a designated poultry house with an attached run area.

Housing

- **Poultry House:** A shelter where birds are housed at night to protect them from predators and harsh weather conditions.
- **Run:** An enclosed area adjacent to the poultry house, surrounded by wire mesh, where birds can roam freely during the day.

Space Requirements

- **Poultry House:** Approximately 3-4 square feet per bird.
- **Run Area:** 2m x 2.5m for about 40 birds.

Feeding

- **Primary Source:** Birds forage in the run during the day, supplementing their diet with natural food sources such as insects and plants.
- **Supplementary Feeding:** Additional feed may be provided to ensure the birds meet their nutritional needs.

Management

- **Day time:** Birds have access to the run for foraging and exercise throughout the day.
- **Night time:** Birds are housed in the poultry house to ensure safety and shelter.

Advantages

- **Balance:** Offers a compromise between free range and intensive systems, allowing birds to forage while also providing a controlled environment.
- **Space Utilization:** Provides ample space for birds to roam, promoting natural behaviors and better health.

Disadvantages

- **Space Requirements:** Requires more space and infrastructure compared to the free-range system, which can increase initial setup costs.
- **Management:** May involve more complex management compared to purely free-range systems, especially in maintaining the run area and ensuring adequate nutrition.

Application: Commonly practiced by small-scale producers who seek to balance the benefits of foraging with the security of a controlled housing environment.

3. Folding Unit System

Description: The folding unit system is similar to the semi-intensive system but offers added flexibility through its portability. This system includes a poultry house and an enclosed run, both protected by wire netting.

Design and Management

- The poultry house and run are compact and can be easily moved from one location to another, hence the name "folding unit." This makes it ideal for small-scale operations and urban settings.
- The system is designed to be versatile, allowing it to be placed on various surfaces, including rooftops of houses.

Space Requirements

- **House:** Approximately 1 sq. ft. per bird
- **Run:** Approximately 3 sq. ft. per bird
- **Total Space:** 4 sq. ft. per bird. For instance, a folding unit measuring 20 ft. x 5 ft. can accommodate about 25 birds.

Advantages

- **Portability:** Can be easily relocated, making it adaptable to different environments and seasonal changes.
- **Space Efficiency:** Requires less permanent infrastructure compared to traditional systems, making it suitable for urban or limited-space settings.

Disadvantages

- **Labor Requirement:** Moving the unit requires additional labor, which can be a challenge in terms of manpower and logistics.
- **Limited Capacity:** Primarily suitable for small-scale production due to the compact size of the unit.

4. Intensive System

The intensive system is designed for commercial poultry production and includes

a) Deep litter system and

b) Cage system or battery system

a) Deep Litter System

Description: The deep litter system is a popular method for both small and large-scale commercial poultry farming. It provides a suitable environment for poultry while allowing for easy management and maintenance.

Housing

- **Pen Size:** Each house can accommodate up to 250 birds.
- **Litter Depth:**
- **Broiler House:** 3 inches
- **Layer House:** 6 inches

Litter Materials: Commonly used materials include rice husk, sawdust, wood shavings, chopped straw, dried leaves, and groundnut shells. The choice of litter depends on cost and availability.

Space Requirements

- **Broilers:** Minimum of 1 square foot per bird.
- **Layers:** Minimum of 1.75 square feet per bird.
- **Seasonal Adjustments:** Floor space may be increased during summer months to ensure comfort.

Advantages

- **Ease of Cleaning:** The system simplifies cleaning processes due to the use of litter.
- **Natural Mating:** Facilitates natural mating behaviors among birds.
- **Cost-Effective:** Requires less initial investment compared to some other systems.
- **Comfort:** Provides a more comfortable environment as birds can move freely.
- **Nutritional Benefits:** Litter provides unidentified nutrients, including the "Animal Protein Factor (APF)" (Vitamin B complex).
- **Insulation:** Acts as a valuable insulating agent, maintaining a stable temperature.

Disadvantages

- **Disease Risk:** Higher transmissibility of diseases due to the accumulation of litter.
- **Space Requirements:** Requires more space compared to intensive systems.
- **Feed Consumption:** Less restriction on bird movement can lead to higher feed consumption.
- **Feed Wastage:** Increased feed wastage is common.
- Fertility and Hatchability: Potentially lower fertility and hatchability rates.
- **Disease Incidence:** Higher incidence of litter-borne diseases.
- **Cannibalism:** Increased risk of cannibalism among birds.
- **Egg Quality:** Eggs may become dirty due to contact with the litter.

b) Cage system

Description: The cage system is a modern approach to poultry rearing, optimized for large-scale commercial production. It involves confining birds in cages with minimal space for movement, promoting efficient management and production.

Housing

- **Floor Space Requirements:**
- **Broilers:** 54 square inches per bird
- **Layers:** 60 square inches per bird

Cage Dimensions

- **Breadth:** 1 foot
- **Height:** 1.5 feet
- **Length:** Varies based on the number of birds

Capacity: Ideally, not more than 10-12 birds per cage

Materials: Cages are constructed from strong galvanized wire. A tray is fixed underneath to collect droppings.

Feeding and Drinking: Feeders and drinkers are placed outside the cage to facilitate easy access.

Types

- Californian Type
- Three-Tier Type
- Four-Tier Type

Investment: High initial cost, making it less accessible for small-scale poultry farmers. It is predominantly used in large commercial operations.

Regulations: The European Union banned conventional cages for commercial layer farming in 2012.

Advantages

- **Space Efficiency:** Maximizes use of space.
- **Performance Tracking:** Facilitates easy recording of individual bird performance.
- **Culling:** Simplifies the culling process.
- **Feed Efficiency:** Restricts bird movement, leading to reduced feed consumption and wastage.
- **Disease Management:** No litter, reducing the risk of litter-borne diseases.
- **Disease Spread:** Limited spread of disease due to controlled environment.
- **Cannibalism:** Lower incidence compared to other systems.
- **Egg Quality:** Eggs remain clean, and egg eating is minimized.
- **Fertility and Hatchability:** Generally, better compared to other systems.
- **Litter Management:** Eliminates the cost and management of litter.
- **Energy Expenditure:** Reduces energy expenditure from birds.

Disadvantages

- **Initial Investment:** High cost of setup.
- **Bird Comfort:** Limited movement space makes it uncomfortable for birds.
- **Nutritional Deficiency:** Birds do not obtain unidentified nutrients from litter.
- **Egg Breakage:** Higher risk of egg breakage.
- **Cleaning:** Cleaning can be challenging.
- **Health Issues:** Higher risk of leg problems, cage fatigue, and gangrenous dermatitis.
- **Artificial Insemination:** Often required, demanding additional labor.
- **Welfare Concerns:** Raises concerns about animal welfare.

5. Environmentally Controlled House

Description: The environmentally controlled house is the most sophisticated and modern system of poultry housing, widely adopted in developed countries. It ensures optimal conditions for poultry by maintaining specific temperature, ventilation and humidity levels.

Housing Specifications

- **Temperature:** Maintained at approximately 26°C.
- **Relative Humidity:** Maintained between 50-60%.

  Design:
- **Structure:** Closed building without any windows, oriented longitudinally from east to west.
- **Ventilation:** Equipped with a large exhaust fan on the west side and evaporative cooling pads on the east side.
- **Automation:** Includes automatic feeding and drinking systems.
- **Environment Control:** Ensures proper ventilation, temperature, relative humidity, and lighting.

Production Benefits

- **Feed Conversion Ratio (FCR):** Improved FCR due to optimized conditions.
- **Production:** Enhances overall production and care of birds.
- **Disease Control:** Provides better disease control and safer breeding conditions.

- **Cycle:** Allows for one extra batch (cycle) of broilers to be reared per year.

Advantages

- **Ventilation:** Regulates the ventilation inside the house.
- **Temperature Stability:** Minimizes temperature fluctuations.
- **Humidity Control:** Maintains proper relative humidity.
- **Lighting:** Ensures adequate and proper lighting.
- **Feed Efficiency:** Achieves better FCR in birds.
- **Air Movement:** Provides uniform air movement.
- **Medication Cost:** Lowers the cost of medication.
- **Mortality:** Reduces bird mortality rates.

Disadvantages

- **Initial Cost:** Significantly higher initial investment compared to conventional poultry housing.

Increased energy consumption:

- Maintaining optimal temperature, humidity, and ventilation requires energy-intensive systems, leading to higher electricity bills.

Higher Maintenance and Repair Costs:

- The complex equipment used in these houses can be prone to breakdowns and require specialized maintenance, adding to the operational costs.

Need Trained Skilled Person:

- The operations of Environmentally controlled House need trained and skilled person.

Increased Waste:

- Intensive poultry farming, even with controlled environments, can lead to increased waste generation (manure, dead birds), which needs to be managed properly to prevent environmental pollution.

7

Poultry Housing and its Layout

Mihir Sarma and Rafiqul Islam

Housing of Poultry

Proper housing is essential for successful poultry farming, as it directly impacts the health, welfare, and productivity of the birds. Well-designed poultry housing not only provides protection and comfort but also ensures efficient management and optimal environmental conditions for the flock. This chapter explores the key aspects of poultry housing, including its purpose, site selection, and layout considerations.

Purpose of Poultry Housing

- **Protection and Comfort:** Provides a safe environment that shields birds from predators, harsh weather, and other external threats.
- **Health and Welfare:** Ensures optimal health and well-being by preventing diseases and reducing stress.
- **Management:** Facilitates easy and efficient management of the flock in a controlled and scientific manner.
- **Cost Efficiency:** Reduces overall production costs through efficient resource management.
- **Microclimatic Conditions:** Maintains adequate temperature, humidity, and ventilation, essential for bird comfort and productivity.
- **Performance Maximization:** Enhances flock performance by creating a conducive environment for growth, egg production, and overall health.

Selection of Site for Poultry Farm

1. Accessibility and Market Proximity

- The farm should be situated in a location with easy access to markets for eggs and meat.
- It should also be near suppliers of essential inputs such as feed, chicks, medicines, and vaccines.

2. Transportation Links

- Good road and transportation infrastructure are crucial for efficient movement of products and supplies.

3. Water and Electricity Supply

- Ensure a reliable source of clean drinking water.
- The site should have an uninterrupted electricity supply to support various farm operations.

4. Proximity Considerations

- The farm should not be located near residential or industrial areas to avoid conflicts and potential health hazards.

5. Elevation and Drainage

- Choose a site that is slightly elevated to ensure proper drainage and prevent waterlogging.

6. Exposure to Sunlight and Airflow

- An open site with plenty of sunlight throughout the day and good air movement is ideal for poultry health.

7. Labor Availability

- Ensure the availability of affordable and skilled labor for day-to-day operations.

8. Future Expansion

- The site should have adequate space for potential future expansion of the farm.

Types of Poultry Houses

There are two main types of poultry houses:

A. Open-sided Poultry House

B. Environmentally Controlled Poultry House

C. Open-sided and Poultry Houses

- **Popularity:** These houses are common in India, except in cold and hilly areas, and are known as windowed or conventional houses.
- **Cost and Maintenance:** They are cheaper to construct and easier to maintain.

Construction of Open-sided Poultry Houses

Dimension

- Determined by the number of birds and their space requirements.

- The width should not exceed 9 m to avoid ventilation issues in summer.
- A typical broiler house may be 12 m long and 7.5 m wide, covering 90 sq. m.

Orientation

- In hot regions, the long axis should be east-west to minimize direct sunlight and rainfall.
- In cooler regions, houses should face south or southeast for maximum sunlight exposure.

Length

- Dependent on the number and type of birds.
- Can be any convenient size.

Width

- Should not exceed 12.20 m, preferably 9.0 m.
- For widths over 30 ft., ridge ventilation with proper overhang should be provided.

Plinth

- Should be elevated at least 0.06 to 0.09 m to prevent moisture seepage.

Foundation

- Concrete foundation, with 60 (2 ft) cm below ground and 0.06 to 0.09m above ground.

Height

- Side height should be 7-8 ft, with a center height of 10-12 ft.
- Height in cage houses depends on cage arrangement (3 tier or 4 tier).

Roof

- Preferably gable type.
- Asbestos is ideal for preventing heat radiation, though thatched roofs are an option in low-rainfall areas.
- The roof should have a slope of 1.22 meters (4 ft) for every 3.05 meters (10 ft).

Overhang

- Should not be less than 3.5 ft. to prevent rainwater entry.

Floor

- Should be strong, durable, smooth, easy to clean and disinfect, made of concrete with rat-proofing, and free from dampness.
- Extend 1.5 ft. outside the walls to deter pests.

Floor Type

- Several types are used, including all litter, all slat, slat and litter, wire and litter, and sloping wire floors.
- Choice depends on the grower farm and layer shed requirements.

Side Wall

- Should have a 30 cm half-wall of concrete, with the rest open and fitted with wire mesh.
- The wire nets should be 2.5 x 2.5 cm (1 inch) size of 16-gauge strength.
- Cage houses do not require side walls.

End Walls

- These can be closed from roofline to floor level.

Doors

- Two doors of 6.5 x 3 sq. ft. size, with a foot bath of 1.5x3x0.4 cubic ft. at the entry for disinfectant solution.

Door Step

- Made of concrete, detached by 15 cm (6 inch) from the plinth.

Water Channel

- A channel along the passage saves labor and prevents water spillage, with a proper gradient for even water levels.

Electrification

- Permanent, proper wiring is essential to meet safety standards.

Considerations for House Construction in Winter Weather

- Insulate the roof to reduce heat loss.
- Prefer long houses with 30-40 ft width and several pens to minimize total exposed area, reducing heat loss.
- House should be designed in a way that maximum sunlight enters the shed during daytime.

  Considerations for House construction in hot climate
- House should have good insulation with support of foggers and cooler systems. Increased air movement over the birds by cooler, fan/exhaust to produce wind chill effects which cool birds even without drop in the house temperature. Shed design and construction should not allow direct sunlight inside the house

8

Brooding Management in Poultry

Mihir Sarma and Rafiqul Islam

Brooding is a crucial phase in poultry management that involves the care of day-old chicks during the early stages of their lives. Due to their underdeveloped thermoregulatory systems, chicks cannot maintain their body temperature and thus require external warmth. Proper brooding ensures the healthy growth and development of the chicks. The brooder unit typically includes several key components and considerations.

Brooding of chicks

1. Floor brooding

- Floor brooders (canopy/hover brooder or infra-red bulb brooder) are used to keep specific area(s) within the shed at the desired temperature.
- In canopy or hover brooding method, an umbrella-like canopy with two or three incandescent bulbs (40 to 100 W) each, depending on the season) are fixed at the centre, is inverted and hung in such a way that the birds can move freely in and out of it.
- The bulbs, when put on, heat the air and the hot air is trapped by the canopy preventing the escape of hot air thereby providing warmth to the chicks.
- The height of the brooder should be around 6 inches during the first week.

2. Brooder Guard

- The brooder guard can be made from cardboard, metal sheets, or wire netting. It should be about 18-24 inches in height.
- The guard is placed around the heat source (hover), typically 2-3 feet from its edge.
- The brooder area should be gradually enlarged to provide more floor space, and the guard can be removed completely after 7-10 days.
- A typical brooding unit with four 60-watt bulbs suspended 6 inches above the floor and a brooder guard of 5 feet radius can accommodate 250-300 chicks.

3. Feeders and Drinkers

- For 250-300 chicks, four baby chick drinkers and three brand new egg trays (for feeding) are sufficient initially. These need to be gradually increased as the chicks grow.
- All equipment should be in place, and the brooder should be pre-heated at least 24 hours before the chicks arrive.

Brooding Requirements

- **Temperature:** The optimal temperature during the first week is 90-95°F (35ºC), which should be reduced by 5°F (2.8ºC) each week until reaching room temperature (60-70°F or 21°C) or until the chicks are fully feathered. However, adjustments may be needed based on chick behavior, as their comfort level can vary depending on the local climate.

Table 8.1: Recommended brooding temperature schedule

Age in days/weeks	Brooding temperature
0-7 days/1st week	95°F (35.0°C)
8-14 days/2nd week	90°F (32.2°C)
15-21 days/3rd week	85°F (29.4°C)
22-28 days/4th week	80°F (25.6°C)
29-35 days/5th week	75°F (23.9°C)

- **Ventilation:** Fresh air should be continuously available, but direct wind or drafts should be avoided to prevent chilling. The oxygen and carbon di-oxide concentration should be 21 and 0.3 to 0.5%, while the ammonia concentration should be less than 25ppm.
- **Floor Space:** A minimum of 3-4 inches of floor space per chick is required. Ideally, not more than 500 chicks should be placed under a single brooder.
- **Feeding and Drinking:** Initially, feeds are offered on newspapers or brand new egg trays for the first three days, after which regular chick feeders are introduced. Baby chick drinkers should be provided throughout.

This setup ensures that chicks receive the warmth, nutrition, and care they need for a healthy start to life. Proper brooding management is critical for reducing mortality rates and promoting robust growth in poultry farming.

Preparation of Brooder House

- The brooder house must be thoroughly cleaned and disinfected before the chicks arrive. Use Malathion or Sevin according to the manufacturer's directions, spraying both inside and outside the house (at least 10 feet from ground level). This should be done within 24 hours after the previous flock is removed and before removing litter and equipment.

- Remove all equipment and litter materials from the house after about 48 hours. Clean the house thoroughly, scrubbing all surfaces with brushes and flushing with clean water.
- Soak and scrub the floor and lower parts of the walls with detergent powder and hot water, paying special attention to cracks and crevices.
- Once the building is dry, wash the inside with a disinfectant using a high-pressure sprayer. Suitable disinfectants include solutions of 3-5% cresol or 2-3% caustic soda or lime water.
- Soak and thoroughly clean all equipment, such as feeders and waterers, with a stiff brush, rinse them, and spray them with disinfectant. Sun-dry the equipment for a day.
- Apply a fresh coat of whitewash to the inside walls.
- Spread new litter material throughout the house and return the cleaned equipment.
- Fumigate the house and equipment, using 3X concentration. For conventional houses, close the side walls with curtains before fumigation.
- Provide a foot-bath with a strong disinfectant at the entrance.
- Keep the house locked until two days before the chicks arrive.

Preparation for Brooding

- Spread new, clean, dry, and mold-free litter material on the floor to a thickness of 6-8 cm, depending on environmental conditions.
- Set up the brooding area in the middle of the house, leaving the ends unused. Cover the area with clean, dried gunny bags and then newspapers to prevent chicks from eating the litter.
- Arrange brooders, feeders, and drinkers at least 6-8 hours before the chicks' arrival. Place the canopy (hover brooder) over the newspaper, typically using six 40-watt bulbs per hover for 250 chicks.
- Enclose the brooding area with a brooder guard (18 to 24 inches in height) to prevent the chicks from piling up in corners.
- Turn on the bulbs in the brooder to reach the necessary temperature before the chicks arrive. If needed, cover the nets of the sidewalls and windows with curtains made of gunny bags to conserve heat.
- During winter, use an additional plastic curtain inside the house along with the outside curtains.

- Ensure the brooder and house switches are on to maintain a temperature of 95°F (35°C) at least two hours before the chicks arrive.
- A few hours before the chicks' arrival, fill the waterers so the water reaches room temperature. Boil and cool the water, then mix it with glucose and vitamins.
- Provide feed at least two hours after placing the chicks in the brooder, sprinkling it over the newspaper-covered area within the chick guard.
- After a few hours, transfer the feed to flat-type feeder lids or clean egg trays.

This meticulous preparation ensures that the chicks have a safe and comfortable environment, promoting healthy growth and minimizing the risk of disease.

Feeding of Chicks

- From day-old age to the end of the 6th week, chicks are offered chick feed. Initially, feed should be placed on newspapers/egg trays at least four times a day to encourage eating.
- Before refilling feeders, remove any litter materials and thoroughly mix new feed with any left-over feed. Feeders should be kept full initially, then not more than half full to prevent waste.
- Provide each chick with 5 cm (2 inches) of feeder space and 2.5 cm (1 inch) of water space. Proper feeder height is crucial for accessibility.
- Distribute feeders uniformly throughout the brooder house, ensuring no chick is far from feed. Avoid placing feeders directly under heat sources.
- Once brooders are removed, align feeders parallel to natural light to minimize shadows. Lift one end of feeders before refilling to consolidate leftover feed.
- Ensure adequate feeders are available to prevent crowding and spillage. Maintain proper feeder height throughout the growing period.

Watering of Chicks

- Use lukewarm water, especially during the first four weeks, to reduce chick mortality.
- Waterers should never run dry, as a lack of water can significantly impact growth.
- It is more important to provide ample drinking surface area than to focus solely on the water volume in waterers.
- Multiple small waterers are preferable to a few large ones.

Few Tips for Brooding Management

- Gently place chicks in the brooder. Separate weak chicks and provide them with additional heat as needed.
- Initially, provide fresh water without feed for several hours. An 8% sugar solution with 1% sodium chloride can be given for the first 15 hours.
- In case of stress from travel or weather, add anti-stress medication to the water for the first 3-4 days. Products like Zeetress, Stressban powder, and Stresroak are available for this purpose.
- Ensure all chicks are drinking water. Some may need guidance to drink by dipping their beaks in the water.
- Feed should be immediately offered on the newspaper/egg trays after giving drinking water in the brooder.
- Continuous monitoring, especially during the first few days, is crucial to ensure the chicks' well-being and proper adjustment to their environment.

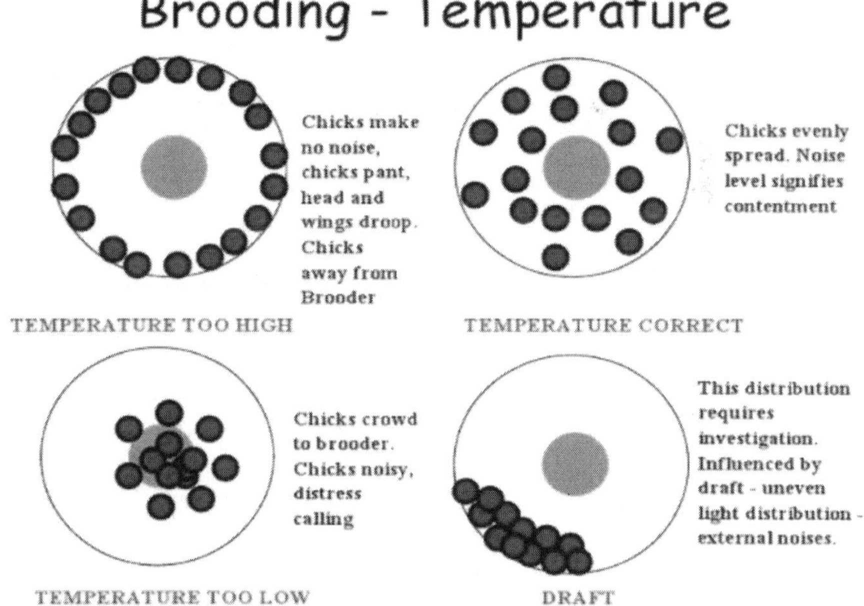

Fig. 8.1: Behaviour of chicks at different brooding temperature

9

Care and Management of Broilers and Layer

Mihir Sarma and Rafiqul Islam

Care and Management of Meat-Type Chickens (Broilers)

Broiler Overview

- Broilers are unisex young chickens raised specifically for meat production. They are typically grown to reach a body weight of 2.0 to 2.5 kg within 5 to 6 weeks, consuming 3.0 to 3.5 kg of feed, resulting in a feed conversion ratio of 1.50 to 1.75.
- Broiler meat is flvored for its tenderness, high-quality protein content, low fat and cholesterol levels, superior flavor, and juiciness.
- The broiler production cycle is divided into three phases based on the birds' physiological and production needs: broiler starter (0-10 days), broiler grower (11-21 days), and broiler finisher (22 days to marketing).

Shed Preparation

- The deep litter system is commonly used in broiler farming.
- An all-in, all-out system is ideal for rearing broilers, although small and medium farmers may not always find this feasible.

Shed Readiness Checklist

- Remove old litter materials and dispose of them properly after the previous batch of birds is removed.
- Thoroughly clean, wash, and disinfect the shed before new chicks arrive.
- Ensure new litter materials are available before starting a new batch.
- Clean, wash, and disinfect all equipment, including feeders and drinkers, from the previous batch.
- Provide appropriate floor space for chicks according to their age.
- Implement a biosecurity plan, including foot baths, well in advance.

Brooding Arrangement

- Start brooding at a temperature of 35°C, gradually reducing it by 2.8°C per week until it matches the environmental temperature.
- Brooding is generally required for 2-3 weeks for broiler chicks, depending on the environmental temperature; cooler conditions require longer brooding periods.
- Monitor brooding temperature frequently, especially during the first 24 hours, and adjust as necessary.
- Observe chick behavior to ensure they receive adequate heat.

Lighting Management

- The primary purpose of lighting in a broiler house is to make feed and water visible to the chicks.
- Provide continuous lighting (24 hours) for broiler chicks, with one hour of darkness each day to acclimatize them to power failures.
- During brooding, use 23 hours of light and 1 hour of darkness to minimize panic huddling.
- Use 10 W bulbs per square meter during brooding and 2.70 W bulbs for the remaining period, with bulbs placed approximately 2.4 m above the floor.

Feeding and Watering Management

- Offer feed on newspaper, egg filler flats, etc., during the first 4-5 days of life, then switch to linear or automatic feeders.
- Feed broiler chicks crumble-form of feed during their first 10 days.
- Broilers are typically fed ad libitum from day-old to marketing.
- Three types of feed are provided: broiler starter feed (BSF) for 1-10 days, broiler grower feed (BGF) for 11-21 days, and broiler finisher feed (BFF) from 22 days to marketing.
- Under standard management conditions, a broiler consumes 3.0 to 3.5 kg of feed up to 6 weeks of age to reach a body weight of 2.0 to 2.2 kg.
- Feed birds twice daily, usually in the morning and evening.
- Ensure adequate feeding and watering space according to the birds' age or size for optimal production.
- Provide sanitized, clean, potable drinking water at all times. Add sugar or glucose to the water on the first day if chicks have been transported for more than 6-8 hours.

- Under normal climatic conditions (21°C), 2 liters of water are required per kg of feed consumed, while in hot climates, 4 liters of water are needed per kg of feed consumed by broilers.
- Feed the birds according to their nutrient requirements (BIS, 2024).

Table 9.1: Nutrient requirement of broiler chicken (BIS, 2024)

Sl. No.	Characteristics	Broiler starter (1-10 days)	Broiler grower (11-21 days)	Broiler finisher (22 days to marketing)
1	Moisture (%) Max	11.0	11.0	11.0
2	Crude protein(%)Min	22.5	21.0	19.5
3	Metabolizableenergy (Kcal/kg)Min	3000	3050	3100
4	Etherextract (%)Min	3.0	3.5	4.0
5	Crude fibre (%) Max	5.0	5.0	5.0
6	Acidinsoluble ash (%) Max	2.5	2.5	2.5
7	Salt(asNaCl) (%)Max	0.5	0.5	0.5
8	Calcium(%)Min	1.0	1.0	1.0
9	Totalphosphorus (%)Min	0.8	0.75	0.70
10	Availablephosphorus (%)Min	0.48	0.46	0.44
12	Lysine (%) Min	1.3	1.2	1.0
13	Methionine (%)Min	0.5	0.5	0.45
14	Vit-A (IU/kg)	11000	11000	11000
15	Vit-B_2 (mg/kg)	6.0	6.0	6.0
16	Vit-D_3 (ICU/kg)	3000	3000	3000

Table 9.2: Expected performance of broiler (Typical Body Weights, Feed Requirements and FCR, Straight Run)

Age (Weeks)	Body weight (g)	Weekly body weight gain (g)	Weekly feed consumption (g)	Cumulative feed consumption (g)	Weekly FCR	Cumulative FCR
1	160	120	124	124	1.04	1.04
2	420	260	317	441	1.22	1.16
3	792	372	530	971	1.44	1.30
4	1260	469	746	1717	1.61	1.41
5	1760	500	904	2622	1.82	1.52
6	2282	522	978	3600	1.95	1.61

Care and Management of Egg-Type Chickens

Egg type chickens (layers) are such types of chickens which are exclusively reared for egg production. They are the key part of commercial egg industry.

They start laying at 19-20 weeks of age and continued up to 72 weeks of age and can produce 300-320 numbers of eggs/ bird.

Management of Egg-Type Chickens (Layers)

The life cycle of egg-type chickens is divided into three distinct phases:

1. Chick Phase (0 to 8 weeks)
2. Grower Phase (9 to 20 weeks)
3. Laying Phase (21 to 72 weeks)

Management of Chicks (0-8 weeks)

Preparation of Brooder House

- **Cleaning and Disinfection:** Thoroughly clean and disinfect the brooder house using Malathion or Sevin as per the manufacturer's instructions. Disinfect the exterior of the house at least 10 feet from ground level within 24 hours after removing the previous batch of birds. Remove all litter and equipment from the brooder house after 48 hours.
- **Thorough Cleaning:** Scrub the entire house with brushes, flush with clean water, and wash the floor and lower walls with detergent and hot water. Pay special attention to cracks and crevices.
- **Disinfection:** Once the building is dry, wash down the entire inside with a disinfectant using a high-pressure sprayer. A solution of 3-5% cresol, 2-3% caustic soda, or lime water is effective.
- **Equipment Cleaning:** Soak feeders, waterers, and other equipment, scrub with a stiff brush, rinse, disinfect, and sun-dry for a day.
- **White Washing:** Apply a fresh coat of whitewash to the inside walls.
- **Litter and Equipment Setup:** Spread new litter and return cleaned equipment to the house. Fumigate with a 3X concentration if using conventional houses, with curtains drawn around the side walls.
- **Biosecurity:** Provide a foot-bath with a strong disinfectant at the entrance. Keep the house locked until two days before chick arrival.

Preparation for Brooding

- **Litter and Brooding Setup:** Spread clean, dry, mold-free litter 6-8 cm thick on the floor, depending on environmental conditions. Set up brooding in the center of the house, covering the area with clean, dry gunny bags and newspapers to prevent chicks from eating the litter.
- **Equipment Arrangement:** Set up brooders, feeders, and drinkers at least 6-8 hours before chick arrival. Position a hover brooder with six

40-watt bulbs for every 250 chicks, encircle with brooder guards (30-50 cm height) to prevent piling.

- **Temperature Control:** Preheat the brooder to 95°F (35°C) at least two hours before chick arrival. Use additional curtains as needed during winter to conserve heat.
- **Water and Feed Preparation:** Prepare waterers with room-temperature water, boiled and cooled, mixed with glucose and vitamins. Provide feed two hours after chicks arrive, initially spreading it on newspapers within the chick guard area. Transition to flat feeders or egg trays after a few hours.

Feeding of Chicks

- **Chick Feed Provision:** Offer chick feed from day-old age until the end of the 8th week.
- **Feeding Frequency:** During the initial weeks, feed should be provided at least four times daily.
- **Cleaning Feeders:** Clean feeders of litter materials before refilling. Mix leftover feed with new feed thoroughly.
- **Feed Levels:** Initially, keep feeders full to encourage eating. Later, maintain feed levels at no more than half full.
- **Feeder and Waterer Space:** Each chick should have 5 cm (2 inches) of feeder space and 2.5 cm (1 inch) of water space.
- **Feeder Placement:** Position feeders at an appropriate height for chicks to eat comfortably. Distribute feeders uniformly throughout the house so chicks always have easy access to feed.
- **Avoiding Heat Sources:** During brooding, do not place feeders directly under heat sources.
- **Light Considerations:** After removing the brooder, align feeders parallel to natural light rays to minimize shadows.
- **Managing Leftover Feed:** Before adding new feed, lift one end of the feeder, preferably away from the light, to concentrate leftover feed near the lighted end.
- **Preventing Crowding and Spillage:** Ensure an adequate number of feeders to prevent crowding and feed spillage. Consistently adjust feeder height throughout the growing period to accommodate the chicks' growth.

Table 9.3: Nutrient requirements for egg type chickens (As per BIS, 2024)

Sl. No.	Characteristics	Nutrient requirement			
		Chick feed	Grower/pre-lay feed	Layer phase I (19-45 wks)	Layer phase II (46-72 wks)
1	Moisture (%) Max	11.0	11.0	11.0	11.0
2	Crude protein(%) Min	20.0	16.0	18.0	16.0
3	Metabolizable energy (Kcal/kg) Min	2800	2500	2600	2400
4	Ether extract (%) Min	2.0	2.0	2.0	2.0
5	Crude fibre (%) Max	7.0	9.0	9.0	10.0
6	Acid insoluble ash (%) Max	4.0	4.0	4.0	4.5
7	Salt (as NaCl) (%) Max	0.5	0.5	0.5	0.5
8	Calcium (%) Min	1.0	1.0 (Grower) 2.0(Pre-layer)	3.75	4.0
9	Total phosphorus (%) Min	0.7	0.65	0.65	0.65
10	Available phosphorus (%) Min	0.45	0.40	0.35	0.33
12	Lysine (%) Min	1.0	0.7	0.7	0.65
13	Methionine (%) Min	0.4	0.35	0.35	0.3
14	Vit-A (IU/kg)	9000	8000	8000	8000
15	Vit-B_2 (mg/kg)	6.0	5.0	7.0	7.0
16	Vit-D_3 (ICU/kg)	1800	1600	1600	1600

Watering of Chicks

- **Temperature and Mortality:** Use lukewarm water throughout the brooding period or at least during the first four weeks to reduce chick mortality.
- **Continuous Availability:** Ensure waterers never run dry, as even a short period without water can slow chick growth.
- **Watering Surface Area:** Prioritize providing ample drinking surface area over the amount of water in the waterers. Multiple small waterers are preferable to fewer large ones.
- **Adjusting Waterers:** Replace waterers with larger ones as the chicks grow.
- **Proximity and Placement:** Position waterers so that chicks never have to walk more than 3 meters (10 ft) to access water, with a maximum distance of 2.5 meters (8 ft) between waterers.

- **Preventing Wet Spots:** Rotate waterer locations to prevent wet spots, which can lead to disease outbreaks.
- **Water Quality:** Ensure fresh, clean, potable water is available at all times.
- **Daily Cleaning:** Wash all waterers thoroughly with a detergent powder every morning before refilling.

Light Management for Chicks

- **Light Requirements:** Adequate light is crucial for chick growth and survival, encompassing both natural sunlight and artificial electric light.
- **Initial Lighting:** Provide 24 hours of continuous light for the first 48 hours after chicks arrive.
- **Ongoing Lighting:** From the third day, maintain 23 hours of continuous light with one hour of darkness daily.
- **Darkness Benefits:** The hour of darkness helps improve growth and accustoms chicks to darkness, reducing panic during power outages. This period typically follows sunset.
- **Lighting Protocol:** Turn off all lights inside and outside the shed during the hour of darkness, then turn them back on after an hour until dawn.

Advantages of Proper Lighting Management

- Promotes rapid learning for eating and drinking.
- Supports proper growth rates.
- Enhances feed conversion efficiency.
- Helps control cannibalism.
- Minimizes chick mortality, especially during the first week of brooding.

Debeaking

- **Definition:** Debeaking involves cutting one-third to half of the upper beak and slightly trimming the lower beak of a chicken.
- **Timing:** The first debeaking is performed when chicks are 7 to 10 days old. A second debeaking may be done between 12 to 14 weeks of age. Debeaking should not be performed after 16 weeks of age.
- **Purpose:** The procedure helps prevent cannibalism, feed wastage, and egg eating during the laying period.
- **Tools:** Electrically operated debeakers are generally preferred over manual ones for precision and efficiency.

- **Post-Procedure Care:** Ensure proper cauterization of the beak to stop bleeding before releasing the bird back into the pen.
- **Preventive Measures:** Administer vitamin K in drinking water 2 to 3 days before debeaking to reduce the risk of bleeding.

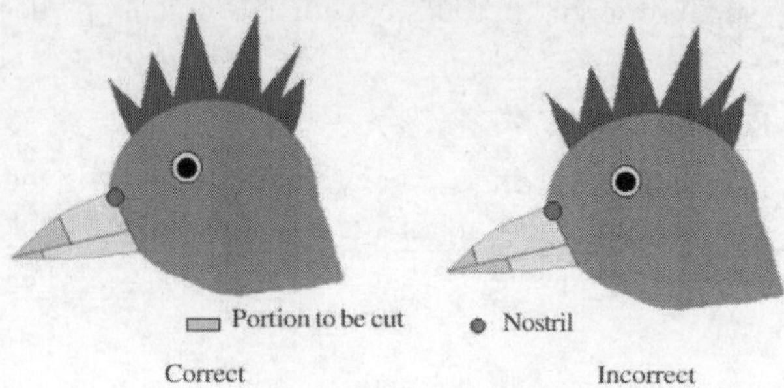

Management of Growers (9-20 weeks)

Housing

- **Deep Litter System:** Grower birds require 1.2 to 1.4 square feet of floor space per bird.
- **Cage System:** In cage systems, the space requirement is 54 square inches (0.38 sq. ft.) per bird. The standard grower cage dimensions are typically 18" width, 15" depth, and 15" height, providing a floor area of 270 square inches, suitable for housing 5 birds from 8 to 16 weeks of age.

Feeding and Watering

- **Grower Feed:** Birds should be fed a specialized grower feed containing 16% protein and 2600 MEKcal/Kg. This feed should be provided until the birds reach approximately 1100 grams in body weight.
- **Feeding Equipment:** Use large longitudinal or hanging feeders for grower birds. Each bird should have 2 inches of feeder space and 1 inch of waterer space in a deep litter system.
- **Water Consumption:** Water intake varies based on factors like ambient temperature, humidity, water temperature, and bird age. Generally, healthy birds drink twice the amount of water as the feed they consume.

Table 9.4: Daily water and feedconsumption of growerat 28°C ambient temperature

Age of birds in weeks	Water consumption/bird/ day (ml)	Feed consumption/bird/ day (g)	Body weight (g)
1	20	11	70
2	28	16	120
3	54	18	170
4	75	25	230
5	105	35	310
6	120	40	410
7	132	44	490
8	144	48	580
9	147	49	660
10	150	50	740
11	153	51	820
12	162	54	900
13	168	56	970
14	174	58	1030
15	180	60	1070
16	186	62	1110
17	189	63	1160
18	198	66	1200
19	225	75	1280
20	246	82	1360

Deworming

- **Prevalence:** Internal parasite (worm) infestation is more common in deep litter systems than in cage systems.
- **Frequency:** Growers in deep litter systems should be dewormed monthly, while in cage systems, deworming can be performed every three months.
- **Common Anthelmintics:** Piperazine and Levamisole are frequently used to treat internal parasites in poultry.

Feed Restriction

- **Purpose:** Feed restriction is used to delay sexual maturity in growing pullets (8-20 weeks) to increase egg production, extend the production life of layers, and prevent excessive body weight gain.
- **Feed Reduction:** Typically, 8 to 10% of the total feed requirement is reduced, resulting in cost savings.

Advantages

- **Cost Savings:** A reduction of 8 to 10% in total feed leads to significant feed cost savings.
- **Increased Egg Production:** Pullets with less fat accumulation produce more eggs.
- **Early Identification of Weaker Birds:** Feed restriction helps identify and cull weaker birds early, saving feed costs and improving overall flock health and livability in the layer house.
- **Heavier Eggs:** Feed-restricted layers tend to produce heavier eggs with better clutch sizes compared to those fed ad libitum.

Disadvantages

- **Delayed Sexual Maturity:** Feed restriction can delay sexual maturity in birds.
- **Reduced Grower House Survivability:** Weaker birds may not survive, leading to lower survivability rates in the grower house.
- **Technical Supervision Required:** Implementing feed restriction requires careful supervision and management.

Method of Feed Restriction

- **Reduction Techniques:** Feed restriction can be achieved by either limiting the total amount of feed intake or diluting the feed with low-nutrient-dense ingredients.
- **Dilution Ingredients:** Ingredients like de-oiled rice bran, rice polish, and wheat bran can be used to dilute the feed.
- **Common Practice:** Quantitative feed restriction is commonly practiced with Leghorn-type laying pullets.

Litter Management

- **Importance:** Proper litter management is crucial in the deep litter system for maintaining a healthy environment for poultry.
- **Litter Quality:** Use fresh, good quality litter materials.
- **Litter Depth:** Spread litter to a height of 3-4 inches.
- **Moisture Content:** Optimal moisture content in the litter should be between 25-30%. Properly managed litter forms a ball that breaks apart when pressed, while wet litter forms a solid ball and dry litter falls apart like powder.

- **Maintenance:** Rake the litter at least twice daily to maintain optimal moisture levels.
- **Avoid Dampness:** Dampness can lead to wet litter, soiled plumage, breast blisters, and ammonia gas build-up.
- **Preventive Measures:** Avoid leaky and overflowing drinkers, and change their position frequently to prevent dampness.
- **Treating Wet Litter:** Use hydrated lime at 1 kg or superphosphate lime at 0.75 kg per 9.3 sq. meters (100 sq. ft.) to treat wet litter.

Selection of Pullets

- **Criteria:** Select healthy pullets with good vigor for egg production.
- **Uniformity:** Pullets should be uniform in size and weight, ideally weighing 1345 to 1360 g at 20 weeks of age.
- **Exclusion:** Avoid selecting pullets with physical deformities such as lameness, blindness, or emaciation.

Transfer of Pullets to the Layer House

- **Preparation:** Clean and disinfect the layer house thoroughly before introducing the pullets.
- **Timing:** Transfer pullets at 16-17 weeks of age to minimize stress by the time they start laying eggs at around 20 weeks.
- **Conditions:** Shift birds during cooler parts of the day, preferably at night.
- **Avoid Stressful Activities:** Refrain from performing activities like vaccination, deworming, or weighing one week before the transfer.

Management of Layers (21-72 Weeks)

Housing

- **Laying Age:** Hybrid egg-laying birds typically start laying eggs at 19-20 weeks of age and continue for 72 weeks or more.
- **Space Requirements:**
  - **Deep Litter System:** Each bird requires 2.5 sq. ft. of floor space.
  - **Cage System:** Each bird requires 60 sq. inches (0.42 sq. ft.) of floor space.
  - **Layer Cage Dimensions:** Typically, 15” width, 12” depth, 15” height at the back, and 17.5” height in front, providing 180 sq. inches of floor area, suitable for three laying birds.

Preparation of the House

- **Cleanliness and Disinfection:** The house should be cleaned, disinfected, and prepared well before the pullets' arrival.
- **Equipment Setup:** Feeders and waterers should be positioned in advance.
- **Ventilation:** Adequate ventilation is crucial, and the house should be insulated or fitted with curtains to protect against extreme temperatures.
- **Laying Nests (Deep Litter System):** Nests should be placed 7-10 days before the start of egg production. There should be one nest for every 4-5 birds, positioned about 30 cm (1 ft) above the floor level along the walls.
- **Egg Handling (Cage System):** Ensure smooth egg roll-out to prevent collisions or breakages.
- **Lighting:** Artificial light should be evenly distributed throughout the house.
- **Nest Bedding:** Use litter material or paddy husks in the nests to prevent egg breakage.

Feeding and Watering of Layers

- **Diet:** Pullets should not receive layer feed until they reach 5% egg production. The feed should contain 18% CP (Crude Protein), 2700 MEKcal/kg energy, 2.75-3.0% calcium, and 0.8-1.0% available phosphorus.
- **Feed Consumption:**
  - **White Leghorns:** 110-115 grams of feed per bird per day.
  - **Brown Egg Layers:** 120-125 grams of feed per bird per day.
- **Water:** Birds must have access to clean, fresh water at all times. Generally, layer birds drink 3-4 times the amount of water compared to their daily feed intake.
- **Feeding and Watering Equipment**
  - **Feeders:** Use a 6 ft linear feeder for every 30 birds or four to five 18-inch diameter circular feeders for 100 birds.
  - **Waterers:** An 18-inch diameter circular waterer is sufficient for 50 layers, and one nipple drinker can serve eight caged layers.

Table 9.5: Expected performances of commercial layer flocks (BIS 2024)

Age in weeks	Production %	Egg/HH (Week)	Egg (HH)	Daily Feed intake(g)
19	5	0.35	0.35	75
20	15	1.05	1.40	80
21	38	2.66	4.06	90
22	64	4.48	8.54	93
23	83	5.60	14.34	96
24	80	6.22	20.55	102
25	92	5.43	26.99	104
26	94	6.57	33.56	106
27	94	6.56	40.12	108
28	95	6.63	46.75	108
29	96	6.69	53.44	109
30	97	6.76	60.20	111
31	97	6.76	66.96	111
32	97	6.76	73.20	115
33	96	6.68	80.40	115
34	96	6.67	87.07	115
35	96	6.67	93.73	114
36	96	6.66	100.39	114
37	95	6.58	106.98	114
38	95	6.58	113.55	113
39	95	6.58	120.13	113
40	95	6.58	126.69	113
41	94	6.59	133.18	113
42	94	6.68	139.66	113
43	94	6.47	146.13	113
44	93	6.40	152.53	113
45	93	6.39	158.92	113
46	93	6.39	165.31	113
47	93	6.38	171.69	113
48	93	6.37	178.06	113
49	92	6.30	184.36	113
50	92	6.29	190.65	112
51	91	6.22	196.87	112
52	90	6.14	203.01	112
53	89	6.07	209.06	112
54	89	6.07	215.15	112
55	89	6.06	221.21	112

56	89	6.06	227.27	112
57	89	6.06	233.33	112
58	86	5.98	239.31	112
59	89	5.98	245.29	112
60	60	5.97	251.26	112
61	68	5.97	257.22	110
62	87	5.90	263.12	110
63	87	5.89	269.02	110
64	86	5.82	274.84	110
65	86	5.81	280.65	110
66	86	5.81	285.46	110
67	85	5.78	292.20	110
68	84	5.66	297.86	110
69	84	5.66	303.52	110
70	83	5.59	309.11	110
71	82	5.52	314.63	110
72	81	5.44	320.07	110

Phase Feeding in Laying Birds

Phase feeding is a nutritional management strategy designed to adjust nutrient intake according to the production stage of laying hens. This method helps reduce feed costs while maintaining optimal egg size and production efficiency. The production cycle of laying hens is divided into three distinct phases, each requiring specific nutritional adjustments.

Phase I (19 to 40 Weeks)

- **Production Level:** Egg production reaches its peak, up to 95%.
- **Body Weight:** Increases from approximately 1350 grams to 1750 grams.
- **Egg Size:** Increases from about 40 grams to 56 grams.
- **Nutritional Requirements:**
  - **Energy:** 2500 ME kcal/kg
  - **Protein:** 17.5% of the diet

Phase II (41 to 60 Weeks)

- **Production Level:** Egg production decreases to around 90%.
- **Energy Requirements:** Reduced to 2450 ME kcal/kg.
- **Protein Requirements:** Reduced to 16% of the diet.

Phase III (61 Weeks to End of Production)

- **Production Level:** Egg production declines further to approximately 80%.
- **Protein Requirements:** Further reduced to 15.5% of the diet.

Benefits of Phase Feeding

- **Cost Efficiency:** Reduces feed costs by adjusting nutrient levels based on production needs.
- **Consistency:** Helps maintain egg size and quality throughout the production cycle.

Note: Nutrient levels provided in the tables referenced (Table ##) should be consulted for specific formulations.

Table 9.6: Nutrient requirements of egg type chicken during different phases

Nutrients	Phase I (19-40 wk.)	Phase II (41-60 wk.)	Phase III (61-72 wk.)
Metabolizable energy kcal/kg	2500	2450	2450
Crude protein % (min.)	17.50	16.00	15.50
Methionine % (min.)	0.40	0.30	0.30
Lysine % (min.)	0.80	0.70	0.70
Calcium % (min.)	3.60	4.00	4.00
Available Phosphorous % (min.)	0.35	0.30	0.30

Lighting Management

- **Role of Light:** Light plays a crucial role in regulating the reproductive system of poultry. It influences the age at which hens begin laying eggs and the total egg production during a laying period.
- **Natural Day Length Influence:**
  - **Spring:** Increasing day length stimulates sexual maturity and egg production.
  - **Autumn:** Decreasing day length delays sexual maturity and reduces egg production.
- **Adjusting Light Period**
  - **Gradual Increase:** Increase the day length gradually to a maximum of 16 hours, preferably by ½ hour per week, to avoid sudden changes.
  - **Intensity and Distribution:** Ensure proper light intensity (1 watt per 4 sq. feet or 5 to 10 lux) and even distribution throughout the poultry house.

- **Positioning:** Place bulbs 8 feet above the floor and use reflectors to direct light towards the birds. Regularly check and clean the bulbs.

Collection of Eggs

- **Frequency:** Collect eggs four times a day to maintain quality and minimize damage.
    - **Timing:** Collection should be done at 9 AM, 12 PM, 2 PM, and 4 PM.
- **Handling:** Use egg trays or bamboo baskets to collect eggs to prevent damage.

Culling of Poor Layers

- **Purpose:** Culling involves removing unproductive or poor-producing hens to reduce feed costs and improve overall flock performance.
- **Indicators of Poor Layers:** Poor layers often exhibit
    - Reduced activity and alertness
    - Lack of vigor
    - Excessive body fat
    - Loose or poorly maintained feathers
    - Deviations from normal characteristics

By adhering to these practices, poultry management can enhance productivity, reduce costs, and ensure the overall health and efficiency of the flock.

Moulting

Moulting is the natural physiological process where a bird sheds and renews its feathers, typically occurring at the end of its first year of laying.

- **Triggers:**
    - **Hormonal Changes:** Hormones secreted by the thyroid gland.
    - **Laying Cycle:** Completion of a full laying cycle.
    - **Day Length:** Reduction in day length.
- **Timing:** Commercial layers generally moult around 16-17 months of age.
- **Indicators of Layer Quality:**
    - **Good Layers :**Moulting occurs later and is completed more quickly.
    - **Poor Layers:** Moulting occurs earlier and takes longer to complete.

Broodiness

Broodiness is a natural behavior where a hen stops laying eggs and becomes overly inclined to sit on a nest, often leading to a reluctance to leave the nest box.

- **Characteristics of Broody Birds:**
  - **Behavior:** Will sit in the nest box and resist leaving unless forced.
  - **Commercial Impact:** Broody birds are non-layers and are thus culled in commercial operations.
  - **Induction Factors:**
- **Warm Weather:** Can trigger broodiness.
- **Egg Accumulation:** Eggs left to accumulate in the nest box.
- **Reduced Light Exposure:** Less exposure to light.
- **Presence of Chicks:** Exposure to baby chicks can induce broodiness.
- **Biological Mechanism:**
  - **Prolactin Secretion:** The presence of baby chicks increases plasma prolactin levels, which maintains incubation behavior.

By managing moulting and broodiness effectively, poultry producers can ensure consistent egg production and overall flock efficiency.

10

Breeder Flock Management

Rafiqul Islam and Mihir Sarma

Introduction

The performance of any commercial stock (offspring) depends on the careful selection and scientific breeding of their parent stocks, known as "breeders." Breeders are the backbone of any commercial poultry operation, as they produce the next generation of chickens, ensuring the continuity and quality of the flock. A breeder farm's primary purpose is to produce a high number of fertile eggs per layer bird and to increase hatchability through proper hygienic handling of these eggs. Effective breeder farm management encompasses several key areas, including:

- **Pure Line Management:** Focusing on maintaining and improving specific genetic lines.
- **Parent Stock Management:** Managing the birds that directly produce commercial layers or broilers.
- **Grandparent Stock Management:** Managing the generation that produces parent stock, critical for maintaining genetic diversity and quality.

This chapter provides a comprehensive overview of the crucial aspects of breeder flock management, including selection, housing, nutrition, health management, mating systems, egg collection, and record keeping.

1. Selection of Breeders

Genetic Quality

- Select breeders from lines with high productivity, good feed conversion ratios, and disease resistance. Genetic improvement targets traits like egg production, growth rate, and overall vitality.
- For instance, selection criteria may include birds that lay over 280 eggs annually, possess a feed conversion ratio (FCR) of less than 2:1 for layers, or show rapid growth and high meat yield for broilers.

Physical Health

- Breeders should be free from physical defects, such as beak deformities or skeletal issues, ensuring they can thrive and reproduce effectively.
- Healthy breeders exhibit strong legs, clear eyes, and vibrant plumage.

Uniformity

- Uniformity in size and weight among breeders simplifies management and ensures consistent production. Regular monitoring helps maintain uniformity, with layers typically weighing around 1.5 kg at 20 weeks, and broilers reaching 2.5 kg or more.

2. Housing

Space Requirements

- Adequate space is critical to prevent overcrowding, which can lead to stress and reduced fertility. Recommended space for floor-reared breeders is 3-4 sq. ft. per bird, while caged birds require at least 0.75 sq. ft. (112 sq. inches).
- Proper spacing contributes to a healthy environment, supporting better growth and egg production.

Ventilation

- Good ventilation removes excess moisture and ammonia, critical for respiratory health. High ammonia levels (>25 ppm) can compromise bird health and productivity.
- Ventilation systems should ensure at least four air exchanges per hour.

Lighting

- Lighting impacts reproductive cycles, influencing the timing and quantity of egg production. A gradual increase in light duration, starting at 12 hours per day and reaching 16 hours by 20 weeks, stimulates egg production.
- Maintain light intensity around 5-10 lux, with even distribution throughout the house.

Nesting

- In deep litter systems, provide one nest per 4-5 hens, positioned 1 foot above the floor with clean, dry bedding to prevent egg breakage.
- In cage systems, ensure eggs roll out smoothly without damage.

3. Nutrition and Feeding

Balanced Diet

- A well-formulated breeder diet is essential for optimal reproductive performance. Breeder feeds typically contain 16-17% crude protein (CP), 2.75-3.0% calcium, and 0.4-0.5% phosphorus.
- Energy content should be around 2,800-2,900 kcal/kg for layers and 3,200-3,300 kcal/kg for broilers.

Feed Restriction

- Implement feed restriction to manage body weight and optimize fertility. Overfeeding can lead to obesity, reducing egg production and fertility.
- Restrict feed intake by 10-15% compared to ad libitum feeding.

Water

- Ensure constant access to clean, fresh water, with water consumption typically 1.5 to 2 times feed intake, depending on temperature and age.

4. Health Management

Biosecurity

- Implement stringent biosecurity measures, including controlled access, regular disinfection, and protective clothing to prevent disease spread.
- Quarantine new birds for at least 30 days before introducing them to the main flock.

Vaccination

- Follow a comprehensive vaccination schedule based on local disease prevalence. Key vaccines include those for Newcastle Disease, Infectious Bronchitis, Marek's Disease, and Avian Influenza.
- Regular health checks and serological monitoring help assess flock immunity.

Regular Health Checks

- Conduct routine inspections for signs of illness, such as changes in behavior or abnormal droppings. Isolate and treat sick birds promptly.

5. Mating Management

Male to Female Ratio

- Maintain an optimal male-to-female ratio, typically 1:10 for commercial layers and 1:8 for broilers, to ensure high fertility rates.
- Adjust the ratio based on fertility monitoring.

Artificial Insemination (AI)

- AI can enhance genetic diversity and ensure high fertility, especially in large or valuable flocks.
- AI is performed every 4-7 days, depending on breed and fertility needs.

Mating Systems

The mating system used in breeder flock management plays a critical role in ensuring high fertility rates and maintaining the genetic quality of the flock. The choice of mating system depends on factors such as flock size, breeding goals, and available resources. The main mating systems used in poultry breeding include:

Pen Mating

- **Description:** In pen mating, a specific number of males are housed with a specific number of females in a pen. This system allows for some level of individual bird management and control over mating pairs.
- **Advantages:**
  - Easier to manage and monitor mating activities.
  - Reduces the risk of over-mating or under-mating.
  - Suitable for small to medium-sized flocks.
- **Disadvantages:**
  - Requires more space and infrastructure.
  - Limited genetic diversity as the same males are used repeatedly.

Flock Mating

- **Description:** In flock mating, a large number of males and females are housed together in a communal area. This system allows for natural mating behaviors and is commonly used in large commercial operations.
- **Advantages:**
  - Simplifies management as there is less need for individual bird monitoring.
  - Promotes genetic diversity as multiple males have access to the females.
  - Cost-effective for large flocks.
- **Disadvantages:**
  - Difficult to control individual mating pairs.
  - Risk of over-mating certain females, leading to stress and reduced fertility.
  - Increased risk of injury and disease spread due to high bird density.

Stud Mating

- **Description:** In stud mating, selected males are used to inseminate a group of females either through natural mating or artificial insemination (AI). This system is particularly useful for breeding programs focused on genetic improvement.
- **Advantages:**
  - Allows for precise genetic control and selection.
  - Can maximize the use of superior males.
  - Reduces the risk of over-mating and injury.
- **Disadvantages:**
  - Requires more labor and expertise, especially if AI is used.
  - Higher costs due to specialized equipment and handling.
  - Limited natural mating behavior.

Each mating system has its own set of benefits and challenges. The choice of system should align with the breeding objectives, whether it is maximizing fertility, improving specific traits, or maintaining genetic diversity. For instance, in commercial broiler operations where rapid growth and high feed efficiency are prioritized, flock mating might be preferred due to its efficiency and cost-effectiveness. In contrast, stud mating may be ideal for specialized breeding programs focusing on genetic improvements or maintaining pure lines.

6. Egg Collection and Handling

Frequent Collection

- Collect eggs at least four times daily to minimize contamination and breakage. First collection at 9 AM, followed by subsequent collections throughout the day.
- Regular collection reduces egg eating and ensures clean, fresh eggs.

Sanitation

- Sanitize eggs before incubation using UV light or chemical disinfectants.
- Store eggs at 10-12°C and 70-80% relative humidity to maintain hatchability.

Storage

- Avoid storing eggs for more than 7 days before incubation, as hatchability declines with longer storage.

7. Record Keeping

Data Management

- Keep accurate records of performance metrics, including egg production, fertility, hatchability, feed consumption, and health.
- Document vaccination schedules, biosecurity measures, and treatments.

Analysis

- Analyze data regularly to identify trends and inform breeding and management decisions.
- Monitor key performance indicators (KPIs) like FCR, egg weight, and hatchability.

8. Culling

Criteria

- Cull underperforming or unhealthy birds, focusing on those with physical deformities, low productivity, or health issues.
- Regular culling helps maintain overall flock health and productivity.

Timing

- Cull promptly to reduce economic impact and optimize production.

9. Environmental Control

Temperature and Humidity

- Maintain optimal temperatures (18-24°C for layers, slightly warmer for broilers) and humidity (60-70%) for bird comfort and performance.

Seasonal Management

- Adjust practices for seasonal variations, such as additional heating or cooling as needed.

10. Breeding Objectives

Production Goals

- Define clear breeding objectives, such as enhancing egg production, meat quality, or disease resistance.
- Set specific targets for traits like egg number, egg weight, and growth rate.

Selection Programs

- Implement selection programs based on genetic and phenotypic traits. Use genetic markers and performance testing for effective selection.

- Update breeding strategies regularly based on market demands and technological advancements.

Breeder flock management involves a blend of genetic selection, optimal environmental conditions, and vigilant health monitoring. By adhering to these guidelines, poultry producers can maximize the performance and profitability of their breeder flocks.

Table 10.1: Floor, feeder, and waterer space requirements in breeder chicken (North and Bell, 1990; Sreenivasaiah, 2006)

Type	Floor space (cm²/bird)			Feeder space (cm/bird)		Waterer space (cm/bird)		
	Brooder	**Grower**	**Layer**	**Grower**	**Layer**	**Brooder**	**Grower**	**Layer**
Standard leghorn (all litter system)								
Breeder pullets	790	1600	1900	6.4	9.40	1.50	1.90	2.50
Breeder cockerels	930	1600	1900	7.6	9.40			
Medium size (all litter system)								
Breeder pullets	930	1800	2100	7.6	10.6	2.20		
Breeder cockerels	930	2000	2100	8.9	10.6			
Meat type (all litter system)								
Breeder pullets	930	2300	2800	15.0	15.0	1.9	2.5	3.1
Breeder cockerels	1160	2800	2800	20.0	15.0	2.5	3.2	
Cage system								
Standard leghorn	155	290	389	4.1	7.6	1.9	2.5	3.8
Medium size	181	348	452	6.9	8.4	2.0	3.1	4.3

Table 10.2: Nutrient requirements for breeder chicken (B.I.S. Chicken: IS 1374: 2024)

Nutrient	Broiler Breeder				Layer Breeder			
	Chick	Grower/ Pre-layer	Layer	Male	Chick	Grower/ Pre-layer	Layer	Male
Moisture % (max.)	11.0	11.0	11.0	11.0	11.0	11.0	11.0	11.0
CP % (min.)	20.0	16.0	16.0	14.0	20.0	16.0	17.0	16.0
EE % (min.)	2.5	2.5	2.5	2.5	2.0	2.0	2.0	2.0
CF % (max.)	7.0	9.0	9.0	9.0	7.0	9.0	9.0	9.0
AIA % (max.)	4.0	4.0	4.0	4.0	2.5	2.5	2.5	2.5
Salt % (max.)	0.5	0.5	0.5	0.5	0.5	0.5	0.5	0.5
Calcium % (min.)	1.0	1.0 (grower) 2.0 (pre- layer)	3.5	1.0	1.0	1.0 (grower) 2.0 (pre- layer)	3.8	1.0
Available phosphorus % (min.)	0.45	0.45	0.40	0.40	0.45	0.40	0.35	0.40
Lysine % (min.)	1.0	0.8	0.85	0.8	0.95	0.7	0.7	0.8
Methionine % (min.)	0.45	0.4	0.45	0.4	0.4	0.4	0.4	0.4
Methionine + Cysteine % (min.)	0.52	0.50	0.55	0.50	0.65	0.59	0.65	0.65
ME (Kcal/ kg) (min.)	2800	2650	2700	2750	2800	2600	2600	2600
Manganese, mg/kg (min.)	100.0	100.0	100.0	100.0	100.0	100.0	100.0	100.0
Zinc, mg/kg (min.)	80.0	80.0	80.0	80.0	80.0	80.0	80.0	80.0
Selenium, mg/kg (min.)	0.15	0.15	0.20	0.15	0.15	0.15	0.20	0.15
Vitamin A, IU/kg (min.)	12000	12000	15000	12000	12000	12000	15000	12000
Vitamin D_3, IU/kg (min.)	2500	2500	3000	2500	2500	2500	3000	2500
Vitamin E, mg/kg (min.)	20.0	20.0	50.0	20.0	20.0	20.0	50.0	20.0
Vitamin K_3, mg/kg (min.)	2.0	2.0	3.0	2.0	2.0	2.0	3.0	2.0
Thiamine, mg/kg (min.)	5.0	5.0	6.0	5.0	5.0	5.0	6.0	5.0
Pantothenic acid, mg/kg (min.)	15.0	15.0	25.0	15.0	15.0	15.0	25.0	15.0
Biotin, mg/kg (min.)	0.20	0.20	0.20	0.20	0.20	0.20	0.20	0.20
Vitamin B_{12}, mg/kg (min.)	0.025	0.025	0.030	0.025	0.025	0.025	0.030	0.025

11

Feeds and Feeding Management in Poultry

Ashim Kumar Saikia and Rafiqul Islam

Feeds and Feeding of Poultry

Proper feeding is crucial for the optimal growth, health, and productivity of poultry. It constitutes a significant portion of the total production cost in poultry farming, often accounting for 70-75%. Understanding the different types of feed ingredients and their nutritional contributions is essential for formulating balanced diets that meet the specific needs of poultry at various stages of growth and production.

Different Feed Ingredients Used in Poultry

Poultry feed ingredients are broadly classified into four categories: energy-rich feedstuffs, protein-rich feedstuffs, vitamin and mineral sources, and non-nutritive feed additives. Typically, commercial poultry feeds are formulated by blending 10-15 different ingredients to provide a balanced diet that meets the nutritional requirements of the birds.

1. **Energy-Rich Feedstuffs** These ingredients form the bulk of poultry diets, providing essential carbohydrates and fats necessary for energy. They make up about 45 to 65 percent of the poultry feed composition.

Table 11.1: Commonly used energy rich feed ingredients

Ingredient	Description
Maize Grain	A primary energy source, highly digestible, and rich in carbohydrates.
Jowar Grain (Sorghum)	Similar to maize, it is used extensively for its energy content.
Millets (Bajra/Pearl Millet, Ragi)	Alternative energy sources, often used in regions where maize is not abundantly available.
Oats and Wheat	Provide energy and some protein.
Wheat Bran	A by-product of wheat milling, it is a good source of fiber and energy.
Broken Rice/Rice Kani	A cost-effective energy source, especially in regions with rice cultivation.
Rice Bran and Rice Polish	By-products of rice milling, rich in energy and also contain some protein.
Salseed Cake	An unconventional energy source, used in limited amounts due to its anti-nutritional factors.
Tapioca Flour	A starch-rich ingredient used for energy.
Molasses	Primarily used for energy, also acts as a binder in pellet feed.

2. **Protein-Rich Feedstuffs** These ingredients are essential for growth, feather development, egg production, and overall health. They are categorized into vegetable and animal protein sources.

Table 11.2: Commonly used protein rich feed ingredients

Type	Ingredient	Description
Vegetable Protein Sources	Groundnut Cake	A widely used protein source, rich in essential amino acids.
	Linseed Cake and Sesame (Hl) Cake	Good protein sources but should be used with caution due to possible anti-nutritional factors.
	Sunflower Cake and Mustard Cake	Commonly used in poultry diets for their protein content.
	Cotton Seed Cake	Used sparingly due to gossypol, a toxic compound.
	Soybean Cake	Highly valued for its high-quality protein and balanced amino acid profile.
	Coconut Cake	A by-product of oil extraction, used as a protein source.
	Maize Gluten Meal	A by-product of maize processing, rich in protein.
	Guar Meal	Contains protein and can be used as a partial substitute for more expensive protein sources.
	Penicillium-Mycelium Waste	An unconventional protein source derived from industrial processes.

Animal Protein Sources	Fish Meal	Rich in essential amino acids and minerals, particularly calcium and phosphorus.
	Meat Meal and Blood Meal	By-products of the meat industry, rich in protein and minerals.
	Liver Residue Meal	Provides high-quality protein and essential vitamins.
	Silk Worm Pupae Meal	A rich protein source with a good amino acid profile.
	Poultry Hatchery By-product Meal	Includes infertile eggs, eggshells, and other hatchery by-products, used as a protein supplement.

3. **Mineral Sources** Minerals are vital for bone development, eggshell formation, and various metabolic processes.

Table 11.3: Commonly used mineral sources

Ingredient	**Description**
Common Salt	Essential for maintaining electrolyte balance and osmotic pressure.
Oyster Shell (37.4% Ca)	A calcium source, crucial for eggshell formation.
Lime Stone (37.5% Ca)	Another calcium source, often used in layer diets.
Bone Meal (27% Ca, 12.11% P)	Provides both calcium and phosphorus, essential for bone development.
Di-Calcium Phosphate (23% Ca, 18.1% P)	A rich source of both calcium and phosphorus, used in balanced feed formulations.
Commercial Mineral Mixtures	Available in the market, these provide a balanced supply of essential minerals.

4. **Vitamin Sources** Vitamins are essential for growth, reproduction, and overall health. They can be supplied through natural ingredients or commercial premixes.

Table 11.4: Commonly used vitamin sources

Source	**Description**
Feed Ingredients	Natural sources providing various vitamins depending on the ingredient type.
Commercial Vitamin Mixtures	These mixtures ensure adequate levels of vitamins like A, D, E, K, and B complex vitamins, tailored to poultry needs.

5. **Non-Nutritive Feed Additives** These additives do not provide direct nutritional value but are used to enhance feed efficiency, growth, and health.

Table 11.5: List of non-nutritive feed additives

Additive	Description
Antibiotics	Used as growth promoters and to prevent diseases, though their use is being increasingly regulated.
Coccidiostats	Used to prevent and control coccidiosis, a common parasitic disease in poultry.
Antioxidants	Prevent feed oxidation and spoilage, ensuring feed quality and shelf life.
Antifungals	Prevent mold growth and mycotoxin production in feed.
Anthelmintics	Used to control parasitic worms.
Vitamin Supplements	Additional vitamins to ensure nutritional adequacy.
Antistress Medicines	Help to reduce the impact of stress on poultry, particularly during transport and environmental changes.
Enzymes	Aid in the digestion of specific feed components, improving nutrient availability.

Effective feed and feeding management in poultry involve understanding the nutritional needs of the birds and providing balanced diets with appropriate ingredients. The selection and proportion of feed ingredients directly impact the growth, health, and productivity of the poultry, making it a crucial aspect of successful poultry farming.

Table 11.6: Approximate total feed consumption by different types of poultry

Type of bird	Age of the bird	Type of feed offered	Feed requirement/ bird (Approx.)	
Broiler chicken	1 to 10 days	Broiler starter feed	190 to 200 g	Total feed requirement per bird=3600 g (Approx.)
	11 to 21 days	Broiler grower feed	800 to 1000 g	
	22 to 42 days	Broiler finisher feed	2200 to 2400 g	
Layer chicken	0 to 8 weeks	Chick feed	2.0 kg	Total feed requirement/bird= 47.5 kg (Approx.)
	9 to 20 weeks	Grower feed	5.5 kg	
	21 to 72 weeks	Layer feed	40.0 kg	
Duck (Khaki Campbell)	0 to 2 weeks	Starter feed	0.37 kg	Total feed requirement/duck= 62-63 kg (Approx.)
	3 to 8 weeks	Grower feed (Phase I)	4.11 kg	
	9 to 20 weeks	Grower feed (Phase II)	8.15 kg	
	21 weeks onwards	Layer feed	50 kg	

Quail (Layer)	0 to 3 weeks	Starter mash	85 g
	4 to 5 weeks	Grower mash	250 g
	6 weeks onwards	Layer mash	9300 g Up to 1 year of laying
Quail (Broiler)	3 to 3 weeks	Starter mash	500 g
	4 to 6 weeks	Grower mash	

- These figures are guide only for rearing of laying ducks under complete confinement in intensive system. If the ducks are reared under semi-intensive system with the facility of water source (like pond), feed requirement is very less @ 50-60 g/ adult bird/ day, because they can manage their feed requirement up to 60% from the range land and pond in terms of insects, food grains, grasses, etc.

Feeding systems of poultry

Feeding systems play a crucial role in the overall health, growth, and productivity of poultry. Selecting the right feeding system depends on factors like the type of birds, their age, and the specific production goals, whether for meat or egg production. Various systems have been developed to ensure that birds receive a balanced diet with all the essential nutrients. The main feeding systems include whole grain feeding, grain and mash feeding, all mash feeding, pellet feeding, and crumble feeding. Each system has its unique advantages and challenges, influencing factors such as cost, ease of feeding, nutrient intake, and potential for feed wastage. The table below provides a detailed comparison of these feeding systems, outlining their descriptions, benefits, and drawbacks.

The common systems of feeding poultry are-

1. Whole grain feeding
2. Grain and mash feeding
3. All mash feeding
4. Pellet feeding
5. Crumble feeding

A tabular representation of the different feeding systems used in poultry:

Table 11.7: Different feeding systems used in poultry

Feeding System	Description	Advantages	Disadvantages
Whole Grain Feeding System	Feed ingredients (mainly grains) are offered separately in different containers.	Birds can choose what they want to eat.	Not suitable for commercial purposes; requires more time and labor; birds may not receive all essential nutrients due to selective feeding, leading to deficiencies.
Grain and Mash Feeding System	Both grains and mash are offered in the same container, allowing birds to eat a mixture.	Nutrient levels can be adjusted based on the birds' needs, including growth, egg production, and environmental conditions.	Birds may still selectively feed, leading to potential nutrient deficiencies.
All Mash Feeding System	All feed ingredients are ground to a uniform particle size and mixed as mash; only this feed is offered to the birds.	Prevents selective feeding, ensuring birds receive all nutrients; preferred by most poultry species; wet mash can increase consumption in summer and reduce wastage.	None significant; popular for commercial production.
Pellet Feeding System	Feed is processed into small cylindrical shapes called pellets; the size varies based on the birds' age.	Minimizes selective feeding; ensures even distribution of nutrients, including vitamins and minerals; reduces feed wastage.	More expensive (approximately 10% more costly than mash); less suitable for small-scale production.
Crumble Feeding System	Crumbles are coarser, broken-down pellets.	Easier for young chickens to consume compared to pellets; ensures consistent intake of nutrients without the hardness of pellets.	Similar to pellets, but with finer consistency, making it suitable for younger birds.

This table provides a clear comparison of the various feeding systems, highlighting their descriptions, advantages, and disadvantages.

Table 11.7: Composition of common poultry feed ingredients (on dry matter basis, in per cent), BIS, 2024

Ingredients	ME Kcal/kg	Crude Protein	Crude Fat	Crude Fibre	Total Ash	Sand Silica	Lysine	Methionine	Methionine + Cystine	Tryptophan	Threonine	Linoleic Acid
Energy sources												
Maize	3 300	9	4	2	1.5	1	0.27	0.17	0.37	0.08	0.31	1
Broken rice	2 600	7.9	1.7	1.4	4	2	0.26	0.2	0.27	0.9	0.26	0.6
Jowar	3000	10	3	4	3	1	0.22	0.17	0.38	1	0.31	1.1
Wheat	3 100	14	2.6	2.5	2	1	0.38	0.21	0.5	0.15	0.38	2
Rice polish	2 700	12.7	14	5	8	2.5	0.54	0.24	0.5	0.14	0.53	1
Vegetable fat	8800	-	99.4	9	-	-	-	-	-	-	-	31.0
Protein sources:												
Soy extract	2500	48	1	3.5	5	2	2.98	0.69	1.41	0.61	1.89	0.4
Soy meal	2250	44	0.8	6.5	6	2.5	2.75	0.64	1.31	0.57	1.76	0.4
Groundnut extract	2690	48	1.5	6.8/	7.2	2.5	1.77	0.42	1.15	0.5	1.16	0.19
Groundnut meal	2400	44	1	10	8	2.5	1.39	0.42	1.1	0.41	1.12	0.19
Rapeseed extract	1900	36	1.7	11.5	7	2	2.02	0.73	1.64	0.47	1.58	0
Sunflower extract	1540	28	1	24	7.7	2	1.06	0.67	1.15	0.34	1.05	0.5
DDGS (rice)	2883	46	4.5	4.9	10.2	4.28	1.34	1.13	2.01	0.55	1.66	-
Sesame extract	2200	44	0.5	6.1	11.5	2	1.01	1.16	1.97	0.54	1.44	1.9
Full fat soy	3300	38	18	5	4.6	2	2.37	0.51	1.16	0.69	1.57	7.7
Maize gluten42	3150	42	2	4	3	1.5	0.8	1.0	1.6	0.2	1.1	-
Maize gluten60	3650	60	2	2.5	1.3	0.5	1.1	1.5	2.3	0.3	1.6	-
Fishmeal	2180	45	7	1	22	5	2.5	0.84	1.15	0.7	1.4	-

Meat and bone meal	1848	45	8.6	2.1	38	-	2.48	0.65	1.16	0.29	1.6	0.3
Rice Brandoc	1800	16	0.5	14	12.5	5	0.66	0.31	0.64	0.17	0.54	-
Wheatbran	1400	14.5	3	11	7	2	0.63	0.23	0.56	0.28	0.52	1.7
Salseedextract	2500	9	1	3	-	1.5	0.5	0.32	0.52	0.1	0.3	0.3
Molasses	2000	3	-	-	9.5	-	-	-	-	-	-	-

Table 11.8: Levels of inclusion of common feed ingredients in poultry rations (in per cent)

Sl. No.	Ingredients	Chicks and broilers	Layers
	Energy sources:		
1	Maize	70	70
2	Wheat	20	30
3	Wheat bran	5	10
4	Rice	10	20
5	Broken rice	10	20
6	Rice bran	20	30
7	Rice polish	50	50
8	Fats and oils	5	5
9	Molasses, Cane	2	3
10	Mutton tallow	6	1
	Vegetable protein sources:		
11	Soybean meal	35	25
12	Groundnut cake	50	40
13	Sunflower meal	10	20
14	Rape seed/ Mustard meal	3	5
15	Safflower meal	5	10
16	Sesame/Til cake	10	15
17	Linseed meal	3	5
18	Maize gluten meal	10	20
19	Guar meal	3	5
	Animal protein sources:		
20	Fish meal	10	10
21	Meat meal	5	5
22	Meat-cum-bone meal	5	5
23	Silkworm pupae meal	2	3
24	Feather meal	2	2
25	Blood meal	3	3
	Miscellaneous ingredients:		
26	Bone meal	2	2
27	Limestone	2	6
28	Salt	0.5	0.5

12

Egg Structure Physical and Chemical Composition

Rafiqul Islam and Mihir Sarma

Reproductive Organs of Fowl and Formation of Egg

The reproductive system of a hen is a fascinating and intricate setup designed to produce one of nature's most perfect foods-the egg. Understanding this system requires a look into its two primary components: the ovary and the oviduct.

The Ovary

The ovary is where the magic begins. A hen typically has two ovaries, but in most cases, only the left ovary develops fully and remains functional. The right ovary, although present, becomes rudimentary and non-functional. The left ovary is responsible for the formation of ova, the initial stage of the egg.

Inside the ovary of a hen are approximately 2000 visible yolk-filled ova. These ova are the potential eggs, each waiting to be developed and released. As a hen matures, these ova progress through various stages of development. The transformation from an immature pullet, which has a small, undeveloped oviduct weighing about 1.1 grams, to a mature pullet ready to lay eggs, involves significant changes. By the time a pullet lays her first egg, her oviduct has grown to weigh around 77.2 grams.

The Oviduct

The oviduct is a remarkable tubular structure, approximately 70 centimeters in length in a laying hen. It is divided into five distinct parts, each with its specific function in the process of egg formation. These parts are the infundibulum, magnum, isthmus, uterus, and vagina.

1. **Infundibulum:** The infundibulum is the uppermost part of the oviduct, funnel-shaped, and about 10-11 centimeters long. When a yolk-filled ova is released from the ovary, it is immediately engulfed by the infundibulum. This stage is crucial as it is also the site where fertilization occurs if sperm are present.

2. **Magnum:** Next in line is the magnum, the longest section of the oviduct, stretching 33-36 centimeters. The primary function of the magnum is to add the thick albumen, or egg white, around the yolk. This layer of albumen provides necessary nutrients and protection to the developing embryo (if the egg is fertilized).
3. **Isthmus:** The isthmus follows the magnum and measures about 10.6 centimeters in length. This part of the oviduct is narrower in diameter compared to the magnum. Here, the inner and outer shell membranes are deposited around the albumen, along with some water and minerals. These membranes play a critical role in protecting the egg from bacterial invasion and physical damage.
4. **Uterus:** The uterus, also known as the shell gland, is the fourth part of the oviduct, measuring approximately 10.1 centimeters long. This section is wider and extensible, accommodating the fully formed egg. Within the uterus, the egg acquires its shell, shell color, and bloom. The shell is composed mainly of calcium carbonate, providing a sturdy barrier that protects the contents of the egg. The bloom, or cuticle, is a protective layer that coats the shell, reducing moisture loss and guarding against bacterial contamination.
5. **Vagina:** Finally, the vagina is the last part of the oviduct, about 5 centimeters in length. This section serves as the passageway through which the egg is laid. The vagina opens into the cloaca, a common chamber and outlet for the intestinal, urinary, and reproductive tracts. When the egg is ready to be laid, muscular contractions help to push it out through the cloaca.

The journey of an egg from the ovary to being laid is a complex and meticulously coordinated process, showcasing the remarkable capabilities of a hen's reproductive system. Each part of the oviduct plays a vital role in ensuring that the egg is properly formed, protected, and ready for the external environment. Understanding this process not only highlights the biological marvel of egg formation but also underscores the importance of each component in producing a high-quality egg.

Formation of an Egg

The formation of an egg is a complex and finely tuned process that begins in the ovary and is completed in the oviduct. Here's a step-by-step breakdown of this process:

- **Formation of Yolk:**
    - The ovary is responsible for the formation of the yolk.

    - Once the yolk-filled ova attain its full size, the follicle bursts and the ovum is released in a process called ovulation.
    - Ovulation typically occurs 30-37 minutes after the previous egg is laid.
- **Infundibulum:**
    - The yolk-filled ovum is immediately engulfed by the funnel-shaped infundibulum after ovulation.
    - The yolk takes approximately 15 minutes to pass through the infundibulum.
    - Fertilization, if sperm are present, occurs in the infundibulum (applicable for hatching eggs).
- **Magnum:**
    - The yolk then enters the magnum section, where thick albumen is deposited around it.
    - The albumen is laid down in circles around the yolk.
    - As albumen forms, the yolk rotates and twists the albuminous fibers to form chalazae.
    - This process takes about 3 hours in the magnum.
- **Isthmus:**
    - After the magnum, the yolk with albumen and chalazae descends to the isthmus.
    - In the isthmus, inner and outer shell membranes are added around the albumen.
    - Some water and minerals are also incorporated into the albumen and shell membranes.
    - This process takes approximately 75 minutes.
    - At this stage, the egg has acquired its full size and shape.
- **Uterus:**
    - The egg then moves to the uterus to add its shell, pigment, and bloom (or cuticle).
    - This process takes around 20 hours.
    - As the egg moves through the uterus, a watery secretion is deposited to the albumen, forming the thin albumen.
    - For hens that lay brown eggs, the brown pigments are added to the shell during the last hours of shell formation.

- **Final Stages:**
  - Throughout the egg formation process, the egg passes through the oviduct small end first.
  - Just before laying, the egg rotates and is laid large end first.
  - Oviposition is the act of pushing the egg from the oviduct.
  - The total time to form a new egg is approximately 25 hours and 25 minutes.
- **Formation of Air Cell:**
  - The air cell is not formed at the time of laying but develops as the contents of the egg cool and contract after laying.
  - It usually forms at the broader end between the inner and outer shell membrane.
  - The size of the air cell can help determine the age of an egg.

This detailed process highlights the remarkable efficiency and precision involved in the formation of an egg, showcasing the biological prowess of hens in producing a vital source of nutrition.

Process of egg formation

The formation of an egg is a complex and finely tuned process that begins in the ovary and is completed in the oviduct. Here's a step-by-step breakdown of this process:

- **Formation of Yolk:**
  - The ovary is responsible for the formation of the yolk.
  - Once the yolk-filled ova attain its full size, the follicle bursts and the ovum is released in a process called ovulation.
  - Ovulation typically occurs 30-37 minutes after the previous egg is laid.
- **Infundibulum:**
  - The yolk-filled ovum is immediately engulfed by the funnel-shaped infundibulum after ovulation.
  - The yolk takes approximately 15 minutes to pass through the infundibulum.
  - Fertilization, if sperm are present, occurs in the infundibulum (applicable for hatching eggs).
- **Magnum:**
  - The yolk then enters the magnum section, where thick albumen is deposited around it.

    - The albumen is laid down in circles around the yolk.
    - As albumen forms, the yolk rotates and twists the albuminous fibers to form chalazae.
    - This process takes about 3 hours in the magnum.
- **Isthmus:**
    - After the magnum, the yolk with albumen and chalazae descends to the isthmus.
    - In the isthmus, inner and outer shell membranes are added around the albumen.
    - Some water and minerals are also incorporated into the albumen and shell membranes.
    - This process takes approximately 75 minutes.
    - At this stage, the egg has acquired its full size and shape.
- **Uterus:**
    - The egg then moves to the uterus to add its shell, pigment, and bloom (or cuticle).
    - This process takes around 20 hours.
    - As the egg moves through the uterus, a watery secretion is deposited to the albumen, forming the thin albumen.
    - For hens that lay brown eggs, the brown pigments are added to the shell during the last hours of shell formation.
- **Final Stages:**
    - Throughout the egg formation process, the egg passes through the oviduct small end first.
    - Just before laying, the egg rotates and is laid large end first.
    - Oviposition is the act of pushing the egg from the oviduct.
    - The total time to form a new egg is approximately 25 hours and 25 minutes.
- **Formation of Air Cell:**
    - The air cell is not formed at the time of laying but develops as the contents of the egg cool and contract after laying.
    - It usually forms at the broader end between the inner and outer shell membrane.
    - The size of the air cell can help determine the age of an egg.

This detailed process highlights the remarkable efficiency and precision involved in the formation of an egg, showcasing the biological prowess of hens in producing a vital source of nutrition.

Details of egg formation

The process of egg formation in hens is a carefully coordinated journey through various parts of the reproductive tract. Each section of the oviduct plays a crucial role in developing the egg's structure and composition. The details of this process are summarized below:

Table 12.1: Different Parts of the Female Reproductive Tract and Their Roles in Egg Formation

Parts of the Oviduct	Approximate Length (cm)	Approximate Time Spent	Activities of Egg Formation
Infundibulum	10-11	15 minutes	Engulfs the yolk-filled ova after ovulation
Magnum	33-36	3 hours	Secretes and deposits thick albumen around the yolk; formation of chalazae
Isthmus	10.6	75 minutes	Adds inner and outer shell membranes around the thick albumen; adds some water and minerals
Uterus	10.1	20 hours 45 minutes	Adds thin albumen around the thick albumen; further addition of shell, pigment, and bloom (cuticle)
Total	63.7-67.7	25 hours 25 minutes	Total time spent in forming a complete egg

This table highlights the intricate and efficient process of egg formation, detailing the specific functions of each part of the oviduct in producing a fully formed egg.

Defects During Egg Formation

Eggs can have defects during formation, including internal and external issues:

Internal Defects: These include blood spots, meat spots, watery whites, pale yolks, mottled yolks, discolored yolks, discolored whites, rotten eggs, roundworms, and off odors and flavors. Blood spots occur when a follicle vessel ruptures during ovulation, while meat spots happen when residual albumen or a piece of follicle membrane from the previous day is incorporated into the egg.

External Defects: These include cracks, pimples, rough, corrugated, and chalky shells, as well as marbling, dots, marks, or weak ends. Pimples are small, raised lumps of calcium on the shell that can feel rough and sandpaper-like. Wrinkled eggs have thinly creased or wrinkled shells, which can be caused by stress, disease, or defective shell glands.

Table 12.2: Common defects of egg during formation

Defect	Cause	Description
Double-Yolked Egg	- Simultaneous release of two yolk-filled ova during ovulation. - One yolk is lost in the body cavity and picked up the next day along with the new ovum.	- Two yolk-filled ova enter the shell gland together to form a double-yolked egg.
An Egg Within an Egg	- Reversal direction of the egg by the wall of the oviduct.	- One day's egg is added to the next day's egg, and the shell forms around both.
Blood Spots	- Rupture of tiny blood vessels in the ovary during ovulation. - Vitamin K deficiency.	- Blood spots are usually found in and around the yolk. - Freshly laid eggs have cloudy albumen, making detection during candling difficult.
Meat Spots	- Residual albumen or a piece of follicle membrane from the previous day. - Varies according to the strain and age of the bird.	- Brown in color and associated with the albumen.
Soft-Shelled Eggs	- Prematurely laid egg with insufficient time in the uterus for shell deposition.	- Results in a soft-shelled egg.
Thin-Shelled Eggs	- Heredity, lack of calcium, phosphorus, manganese, Vitamin D3 in the diet. - Diseases such as Ranikhet disease, egg drop syndrome, etc.	- Results in thin, porous, and sometimes shell-less eggs.
Glassy and Chalky Shells	- Malfunction of the uterus of the laying bird.	- Glassy eggs are less porous and will not hatch but may retain other quality aspects.
Pimples	- Excess calcium deposition.	- Small, raised lumps of calcium on the shell that can feel rough and sandpaper-like.
Wrinkled Eggs	- Stress, disease, or defective shell glands.	- Thinly creased or wrinkled shells.
Off-Colored Yolk	- Lack of pigment substances in the feed.	- Results in an off-colored yolk.
Off-Flavored Egg	- Certain feed ingredients or improper storage of the egg.	- Results in an off-flavored egg.

Physical Structure

An egg consists of approximately 12% shell, 58% albumen, and 30% yolk. However, the physical composition varies with the breed, age, and nutrition of the birds.

Table 12.3: Composition of different parts of egg with their role

Part	Description	Composition	Role
Cuticle	Outermost coating of an egg, also called bloom. Soluble in water and gives a shiny appearance to the shell.	Glycoproteins (mainly) Carbohydrates Fats	Protects against microbial contamination.
Shell	Outermost part, composed of two protective layers with numerous pores (6,000 to 10,000). Contains calcium carbonate.	Calcium carbonate (93%) Magnesium carbonate (1%) Calcium phosphate (1%) Organic matter (4%) Moisture (1%)	Provides structural integrity, allows gas exchange, and contains calcium for embryo development.
Shell Membrane	Two membranes (inner and outer) between egg shell and egg albumen. Flexible when moist, brittle when dried. Composed of protein fibers.	Protein fibres (mainly collagen type I) Glycosaminoglycans (e.g., dermatan sulphate, chondroitin sulphate) Sulphated glycoproteins (e.g., glucosamine)	Provides protection against bacterial invasion.
Albumen (White)	Clear, translucent, colorless, and viscous gel-like mass. Consists of two layers: thin albumen (24%) and thick albumen (34%).	Ovalbumin (54%) Conalbumin (13%) Ovomucoid (11%) Lysozyme (3.5%) Globulins (8%) Ovomucin (1.5%)	Provides protein and water necessary for embryo development, contains antimicrobial proteins.
Yolk	Yellowish mass surrounded by the vitelline membrane. Makes up approximately one-third of the egg's weight. Contains the germinal disc.	Lipids (approx. 33%) Proteins (approx. 16%) Carotenoids (xanthophylls and carotene) Water (approx. 50%)	Nutrient-rich food source for the developing embryo.
Germinal Disc	Reproductive nucleus, also called the germ spot. Enclosed in the vitelline membrane. Diameter is 3.5 mm in infertile eggs and 4.5 mm in fertile eggs.	- Organic matter (protein and lipids)	Site of fertilization and initial embryo development.

Chemical Composition of Eggs

The chemical composition of eggs is influenced by various factors such as heredity, season, diet, and age. A detailed overview is summarized in the table below:

Table 12.4: Chemical Composition of Eggs

Attribute	Details
Average Weight	Approximately 55 grams for a White Leghorn egg
Major Constituents	Water,protein,lipid,carbohydrates,free of fibers
Minerals	94% in eggshell;remaining distributed between egg white and yolk, mostly conjugated forms - Calcium: over 98% of shell minerals - Other minerals: phosphorus, magnesium, iron, sulfur - Yolk: 2% minerals, primarily phosphorus (61% in phospholipids)-- Egg white: Sulfur, potassium, sodium, chlorine
Energy Content (per 100 grams)	- Chicken egg: 143 kcal - Quail egg: 158 kcal - Duck egg: 185 kcal - Goose egg: 185 kcal - Turkey egg: 171 kcal
Lipid Proportion	Approximately 13% across different avian species
Lipid Proportion	- Chicken egg: 9.5% - Duck and - Goose eggs: over 13%
Egg Composition	- Duck and goose eggs have higher fat content and a higher percentage of yolk compared to chicken eggs
Vitamin C	- Eggs do not contain Vitamin C

Table 12.5: The chemical composition of hen egg and its components

Egg and its components	Water (%)	Protein (%)	Fat (%)	Carbohydrate (%)	Ash (%)
Whole, raw, freshly laid egg	76.1	12.6	9.5	0.7	1.1
Egg white	87.72	10.82	0.19	0.85	0.42
Egg yolk	55.02	15.50	26.71	1.09	1.68
Source: Retrieved on 04/07/2024 from the Ciqual homepage https://ciqual.anses.fr/(French Agency for Food, Environmental and Occupational Health & Safety. ANSES-CIQUAL					

The major constituents of an egg are as follows:

Table 12.6: Major nutrients of egg

List of constituents	Egg, whole raw, fresh
Energy (Kcal/100g)	143
Protein (g/100g)	12.56
Carbohydrate (g/100g)	0.72
Fat (g/100g)	9.51
Cholesterol (mg/100g)	372

Calcium (mg/100g)	56
Potassium (mg/100g)	138
Vitamin A, Retinol (μg/100g)	160
Vitamin D (μg/100g)	2.0
Vitamin E (mg/100g)	1.05
Choline (mg/100g)	293.8
FA, Saturated (g/100g)	3.126
FA, Monounsaturated (g/100g)	3.658
FA, Polyunsaturated (g/100g)	1.911
Source: Retrieved on 04/07/2024 from the United States Department of Agriculture (USDA), Agricultural Research Service (2014),	

Microbiology of Normal Eggs: A glimpse

Eggs are a vital food source with inherent protective mechanisms that make them relatively less perishable compared to many other foods. The majority of eggs are free from contamination at the time they are laid, with over 90% of eggs being clean from pathogens. The natural defenses of an egg include its hard shell, the underlying shell membranes, and the cuticle, which help prevent microbial entry and spoilage. However, contamination can still occur post-laying, particularly from environmental sources. The primary pathogen of concern is *Salmonella enteritidis*, which can cause gastroenteritis if ingested. This pathogen is rarely transferred through the hen's ovary-affecting fewer than 1% of eggs produced-but can be effectively controlled through thorough cooking, which ensures that the egg white and yolk are fully set. Spoilage organisms such as *Alcaligenes*, *Proteus*, *Pseudomonas*, and certain molds can lead to various forms of egg rot, including green, pink, and black discolorations, but these are typically encountered only in eggs that have been stored for extended periods. The rapid turnover of eggs through market channels means that consumers seldom encounter spoiled eggs. Contamination can also result from environmental factors such as dust, soil, and feces. To maintain egg safety, it is recommended to wash eggs under warm running water using a cloth or brush with unscented dishwashing liquid, being cautious not to allow contact with soil or bacteria during the process. Pathogenic bacteria like *Salmonella*, *Staphylococcus aureus*, and *Clostridium perfringens* are more likely to be found in liquid eggs, often due to human reinfection, rather than in shell eggs. Proper handling and cooking practices are crucial in minimizing the risk of foodborne illnesses associated with eggs.

13

Incubation and Hatchery Operation

Rafiqul Islam and Ashim Kumar Saikia

Incubation is a critical process in poultry farming, involving the hatching of fertile eggs to produce chicks. This process can be carried out by natural or artificial means. Natural incubation involves placing eggs under a broody hen or duck, allowing the mother bird to provide the necessary warmth and conditions for hatching. In contrast, artificial incubation uses machines called incubators to create the ideal environment for the eggs to hatch. The incubation period, which varies among different poultry species, remains consistent within the same species regardless of whether natural or artificial methods are used.

Incubation

- It is simply the production of chicks by hatching fertile eggs either by natural or artificial means.

Table 13.1: Incubation period of different species of poultry:

Sl. No.	Species	Incubation period (Days)
1	Chicken	21 days
2	Duck	28 days
3	Pigeon	17 days
4	Japanese Quail	18 days
5	Muscovy duck	35-37 days
6	Goose	28-34 days
7	Bobwhite quail	23-24 days
8	Turkey	28 days
9	Chukar partridge	23-24 days
10	Pheasants	23-28 days
11	Guineafowl	28 days
12	Emu	52 days
13	Ostrich	42days

Table 13.2: Difference between natural and artificial incubation:

Sl. No.	Natural incubation	Artificial incubation
1	Performed by broody hen or duck	Performed by an artificial machine i.e. incubator
2	Small numbers of chicks (10-15) can be hatched at a time	Large numbers of chicks (as per requirement) can be hatched at a time
3	No investment	Requires a significant initial investment
4	No need for a skilled person; the broody hen manages the process	Needs a skilled person to operate the incubator
5	No need for power supply or kerosene	Requires an uninterrupted supply of power or kerosene
6	Not suitable for commercial purposes when large numbers of chicks are needed	Suitable for commercial purposes, as it can produce large numbers of chicks at a time
7	Achieves high hatchability (80-100%)	Generally, achieves lower hatchability (70-80%)

Care and handling of hatching eggs before setting

Proper care and handling of hatching eggs are of utmost importance to achieve optimum hatchability. If the eggs are not set immediately after collection, they should be handled properly to ensure good results.

Table 13.3: Steps involved in care and handling of hatching eggs

Step	Description
Collection of Eggs	The eggs should be collected frequently and as early as possible after laying. Delays in collection can cause soiled eggs and damage to the eggshell, particularly in deep litter systems.
Fumigation	Eggs should be fumigated before setting in the incubator. Formaldehyde gas is produced by mixing 20g potassium permanganate ($KMnO4$) and 40ml formalin (37.5% formaldehyde) for 100 cubic feet of space (1x concentration) in the fumigating structure.
Storage of Eggs	Before incubation, the eggs need to be stored in a cool, dry, airy space to achieve the best hatchability. The eggs should be stored at a temperature of 12.8 to 18.3°C (preferably 15.6°C) and a relative humidity of 70-75%. Under such conditions, eggs can be stored ideally for 7-10 days (maximum up to 15 days).
Position of the Egg During Storage	While storing, the eggs should be kept broader end up to facilitate proper gas exchange through the air cell.
Turning of Eggs	If the eggs are not incubated within 3-4 days, they need to be turned daily. Turning is done by elevating alternate ends of the egg case or egg flat each day.
Warming of the Eggs	The eggs should be warmed slowly to room temperature before being placed in the incubator.

Selection of hatching eggs

Not all eggs laid by a hen are suitable for hatching. Therefore, it is essential to select appropriate eggs based on the following criteria:

Table 13.4: Criteria for selection of hatching eggs

Criteria	Description
Fertility of Eggs	Eggs selected for hatching must be fertile, as infertile eggs are unable to produce chicks.
Size of the Egg	The eggs should be neither too large nor too small. An egg size of 55-58g is desirable for better quality chicks.
Shape of the Egg	Oval-shaped eggs are preferred over round or elongated ones.
Egg Shell	The shell must have uniform thickness, texture, and color, and should be free of any tints or cracks. Thin-shelled eggs result in lower hatchability. The shell should be clean, sound, and dry.
Deformity of the Egg	Eggs with deformities such as ridges, encrustations, projections, depressions, cracks, or stains should be avoided.
Soiled Egg	Eggs with high soil or dirt on the shell should be discarded. Soil and dirt can be removed by cleaning and washing before setting them in the incubator.
Egg Quality	Freshly laid eggs should not be set in the incubator immediately. Eggs stored for 2-3 days at room temperature after laying provide better hatchability. Eggs with loose or bubbly air cells should be discarded.

By carefully selecting eggs based on these criteria, one can ensure better hatchability and the production of high-quality chicks.

Incubation and hatching requirements

Certain physical conditions are necessary to achieve optimum hatchability, irrespective of the method of incubation. These include temperature, humidity, ventilation, and turning, which are also known as the principles of incubation or ideal requirements for the incubation of eggs.

Table 13.5: Incubation and hatching requirements of various species of poultry

Species	Incubator	Days of incubation (days	Temperature °C (°F)	Relative Humidity (%)	Ventilation (O_2& CO_2 concentration)	Turnings per day	Egg position
Chicken	Setter	1-18	37.7 (99.7)	60	O_2=21% CO_2=0.3-0.5%	24	Broader end up
	Hatcher	19-21	36.7 (98.3)	70		No	Horizontal
Duck	Setter	1-24	37.6 (99.6)	70	O_2=21% CO_2=0.3-0.5%	24	Broader end up
	Hatcher	28-28	37.0 (98.6)	70		No	Horizontal

Japanese quail	Setter	1-14	37.8 (100)	55	O_2=21% CO_2=0.3-0.5%	24	Broader end up
	Hatcher	15-18	37.4(99.3)	70		No	Horizontal

By maintaining these conditions, optimal hatchability for different poultry speciescan be achieved.

Factors effecting fertility

Eggs must be fertile to produce day-old chicks, and the fertility of eggs plays a significant role in the ultimate production of chicks. The hatchability percentage, or the number of chicks hatched from a given number of eggs, primarily depends on fertility. Fertility refers to the fusion of the male sperm and female ovum to form a zygote in the infundibulum of a chicken. Various factors affecting fertility include:

Table 13.6: Factors effecting fertility of eggs

Factor	Effect on Fertility
Breed	Heavier breeds usually have lower fertility due to genetic composition, poor mating ability, and physical incompatibility.
Age of the Bird	Younger birds exhibit better fertility. In males, fertility decreases after the first breeding season; in females, it declines after the first laying season.
Preferential Mating	Preferential mating by males and females can lead to a reduction in fertility.
Male-Female Ratio	Improper ratios cause reduced fertility. Recommended ratios: 1:15-16 (layer breeders), 1:10-12 (broiler breeders), 1:1-2 (Japanese quails).
Climate	Extreme temperatures (too hot or too cold) lower fertility due to reduced mating frequency from male immobility.
Nutritional Factors	Deficiencies in vitamins (A, pantothenic acid, E, biotin) and minerals (Ca, P, Na, Mn, Zn, iodine) lower fertility.
Diseases	Diseases like avian tuberculosis, aspergillosis, coccidiosis, lymphoid leukosis, mycoplasmosis, and infectious bronchitis adversely affect fertility.
Semen Quality	Variations in semen volume, sperm concentration, and successful mating frequency impact fertility.
Condition of Laying Flock	Good laying flocks have better fertility than poor laying flocks.

Factors effecting hatchability

Hatchability refers to the percentage of chicks hatched from a given number of eggs. It can be measured in two ways:

- **Hatchability (%) on the basis of total eggs set:** This includes all eggs placed in the incubator, regardless of fertility.

- **Hatchability (%) on the basis of fertile eggs set:** This measures the percentage of chicks hatched from eggs that were confirmed to be fertile. Hatchability based on fertile eggs is generally higher than when based on total eggs set.

Table 13.7: Factors effecting hatchability of eggs

Factor	Description
Pre-Incubation Storage	- Temperature: 18°C (64°F) - Humidity: 75% - Position: Broader end up - Duration: Store for no more than 7 days
Incubation Conditions	- Temperature: Maintain consistent optimal temperature - Humidity: Proper levels needed -Ventilation: Ensure adequate airflow -Turning: Regular turning required -Position: Correct placement of eggs
Egg Quality	- Shape & Size: Normal shape and size - Shell Quality: Avoid thin or damaged shells - Internal Quality: Avoid poor internal quality
Breed and Strain	Hatchability varies between different breeds, strains, and individual birds
Environmental Temperature	Maintain consistent and appropriate temperatures in the breeder house
Age of the Breeder Flock	Younger flocks generally have better hatchability compared to older flocks

Hatchery operation

For successful hatchery operation, several critical steps must be followed to ensure optimal conditions for egg development and chick hatching. These steps include meticulous cleaning and sanitization of hatching eggs, proper cleaning and disinfection of the incubator, effective fumigation, thorough testing of incubator functions, careful placement of eggs, and adherence to a loading schedule and breeding stock requirements. Regular testing of incubated eggs through candling is essential to identify and manage infertile or non-viable eggs, thereby improving hatchability and overall hatchery efficiency.

Table 13.8: Various steps involved in hatchery operation

Step	**Description**	**Notes**
Cleaning and Sanitization of Hatching Eggs	- Dry Cleaning: Use fine sandpaper or wire wool for lightly soiled eggs - Wet Cleaning: For severely soiled eggs, use 4-5% Dettol or Savlon solution in lukewarm water - Sanitization: Use sanitizers like chlorine dioxide spray, ozone (O_3-100 ppm), quaternary ammonia (200 ppm in lukewarm water), or formaldehyde gas - Common Practice: Chlorine dioxide spray is widely used	Sanitize eggs within 1-2 hours of collection
Cleaning and Disinfection of Incubator	- Initial Cleaning: Clean thoroughly before use - Sanitization: Use 4% washing soda solution, then disinfect with phenyl or Lysol - Loose Fittings: Remove, wash, disinfect separately, and refit before egg loading	Ensures a hygienic environment for eggs
Fumigation of Incubator	- Procedure: Use 20g of $KMnO_4$ in 40ml formalin to produce formaldehyde gas for 100 cubic feet space for 3-4 hours - Safety: Formaldehyde gas is poisonous at 5 ppm; handle with care	Ensure proper ventilation and safety precautions
Testing of Incubator	- Function Check: Test for temperature, humidity, egg turning, and ventilation - Pre-Loading: Run the incubator for at least 24 hours before loading eggs	Confirms incubator is functioning correctly
Placing of Eggs	- Position: Place eggs with the broader end up - Monitoring: Keep a strong vigil for mechanical faults - Adjustment: Avoid frequent opening of the incubator - Humidity Maintenance: Check water levels in containers daily and refill if necessary	Ensures optimal conditions for embryo development
Loading Schedule and Breeding Stock Requirement	- Loading: In large incubators, load one-third of the total capacity every 7-8 days - Breeding Stock: Approximately one-eighth of the incubator capacity in breeding birds - Example: For a 10,000-egg incubator, about 1,250 breeding birds are needed	Helps maintain consistent hatchery operation
Testing of Incubated Eggs	- Candling Days: Perform candling on the 5th or 7th day to discard infertile eggs, and again on the 18th day to discard dead-in-shell eggs - $5^{th}/7^{th}$ Day: Look for spider-like red lines and visible embryo movement - 18th Day: Fertile eggs will show dark appearance and pulsating movement near the air cell	Improves hatchery efficiency by identifying non-viable eggs

Disposal of hatchery wastes

Proper disposal of hatchery wastes is essential for maintaining a clean and efficient hatchery environment while minimizing environmental impact and preventing disease transmission. The following practices should be adhered to:

Table 13.9: Different hatchery wastes and their disposal methods

Waste Type	Collection	Disposal Method	Notes
Eggshells and Egg Residues	- Collect separately from other wastes	- Composting - Processing for animal feed - Treat and dispose according to local regulations	Ensure residues are treated to prevent disease
Dead Embryos and Culls	- Collect promptly to avoid contamination	- Incineration - Deep burial	Follow biosecurity protocols
Cleaning Agents and Chemicals	- Store in appropriate containers	- Dispose according to local hazardous waste regulations	Requires special handling and disposal
Fumigation Byproducts	- Contain properly	- Dispose of as hazardous waste	Prevent environmental contamination
General Waste	- Collect separately (e.g., packaging materials)	- Recycling - Dispose according to local waste management regulations	Separate from contaminated wastes
Sanitization Residues	- Gather used wipes and cleaning cloths	- Incineration - Disposal as non-hazardous waste	Dispose in accordance with local guidelines

Common incubation problems and their remedial measures

Addressing common incubation problems is essential for achieving optimal hatchability and ensuring the health of developing embryos. Various factors can negatively impact incubation outcomes, ranging from issues with fertility and egg handling to environmental conditions and equipment performance. Identifying these problems and implementing effective remedial measures is crucial for improving hatch rates and maintaining a successful hatchery operation. The following table outlines common incubation problems, their causes, and corresponding remedies to help mitigate these issues and enhance overall hatchery efficiency.

Table 13.10: List of trouble shooting during incubation and their remedial measures

Sl. No.	Problems	Causes	Remedies
1.	True infertility	Poor insemination technique	Inseminate more frequently at proper depth with good semen
		Improper insemination of hen; improper male: female ratio	Proper insemination of hen; replace males; maintain proper male: female ratio
		Preferential mating in pen mating	Mate hen with different females
		Non-sterility of males	Replace non-sterile males with sterile males
		Male are not interested in mating	Check for disease, nutrition problems, foot problems, heat stress, social dominance of females; provide a healthy environment for the breeding flock
		Male too old	Use young males, reinforce natural mating with artificial insemination if old, valuable males should be used
2.	Fertile but pre-ovipositional death	Inbred strains	Avoid excessive inbreeding; use young males
		Parthenogenesis in turkeys	Genetic stocks showing higher incidence of parthenogenesis should be avoided
		Eggs washed at a temperature that is too high	Dry clean eggs; eliminate dirty eggs; produce clean eggs; temperature should be low for washing of eggs (110 to 120°F)
3.	Fertile but no embryonic development	Eggs stored in too low temperature	Hatching eggs should be stored at 55 to 68°F (12.8 to 20°C)
4.	Positive development	Improper collection schedule during hot and cold weather	Collect eggs four times a day when temperature inside house or nest exceeds 80°F
5.	Blastoderm without embryo	Improper storage temperature	Hatching eggs should be stored at 55 to 68°F (12.8 to 20°C)

6.	Cystic embryo	Eggs stored too long	Store chicken, duck, goose, quail and pheasant eggs up to 1 week while turkey and partridge eggs up to 2 weeks
		Rough handling or shipping procedures	Handle eggs carefully from time of collection to hatching of chicks
		Diseased flock (*Mycoplasma spp.*, New Castle disease)	Inspect flock for general and specific health conditions and take preventive measures
		Aged or abnormal spermatozoa	Check insemination technique; use young males
		Eggs from inbred flocks	Change male or introduce new genetic stock
		Improper pre-incubation and egg incubation temperature	Do not allow eggs to pre-incubate, eggs should be stored below 80°F (26.6°C) before incubation. Use setter temperature at 99-100°F (37.5 to 37.8°C). Check egg storage temperature
		Eggs from hens housed above 5000 ft (1500 m)	Avoid high altitude or add oxygen to the incubator
7.	Many dead embryos	Improper incubator temperature	Check thermometer for accuracy of temperature; set temperature at 99-100°F (37.5 to 37.8°C).
		Power failure	Provide UPS (generator) compensate power failure
		Improper turning	Eggs should be turned at regular interval @ three to more times a day in the setter
		Eggs from inbred stocks	Avoid inbreeding
		Poor ventilation of hatchery or incubator	Provide proper ventilation for gas exchange
		Diseased or infected eggs	Use eggs from healthy flocks, do not wash eggs with cold water
8.	Embryos die before pipping	Lower setter temperature; relative humidity too high	Maintain 95°F (37.5°C) dry bulb and 86°F (30°C) wet bulb temperature in well-ventilated setter
		Infected eggs	Use eggs from healthy flocks, do not wash eggs with cold water; Wash eggs in water at temperature of 110 to 120°F (43.3 to 48.9°C)
		Poor nutrition of breeder flocks	Check breeder diet; supply required quantity of vitamins and minerals to the breeder diet
		Presence of lethal gene in stocks	Use vigorous strains; avoid inbreeding

9.	Embryos weak and fail to pip or pip weakly	Vitamin E deficiency	Supplement Vitamin E in drinking water @ 48IU of Vitamin E per gallon of drinking water
10.	Many pips stuck to shell	Hatcher relative humidity too low	Maintain 90°F (32.2°C) wet bulb temperature after pipping starts
		Excessive residual albumen caused by high relative humidity and/ or low temperature incubation	Check thermometer and thermostats; monitor temperature and relative humidity
11.	Chicks pipped and dead	Disease	Use disease free stock
		High temperature and low humidity in Hatcher	Check Hatcher temperature and relative humidity
		Nutritional deficiency	Provide balanced feed to the flock
12.	Malposition	Eggs set small end up	Eggs should be set broader end up in the setter
		Improper turning	Eggs should be turned at regular interval @ three to more times a day in the setter
13.	Chicks hatched too early; thin and noisy	Temperature too high during incubation period	Check thermometer; 1°F (0.6°C) in excess of 99.5°F (37.5°C) will result hatch approximately 24 hours early
14.	Chicks hatched late are soft and lethargic (Soggy chicks)	Temperature too low and relative humidity too high during incubation period	Check thermometer; 1°F (0.6°C) below of 99.5°F (37.5°C) will result late hatch
		Old eggs	Set preferably fresh eggs; allow extra times for hatch by setting old eggs early
15.	Sudden losses at any time	Power and equipment failure	Check incubator temperature regularly and rectify it as early as possible
		Mercury spilled in incubator or Hatcher	Check for broken thermometer and thermostats; clean up all spilled mercury immediately
		Improper fumigation;	Do not fumigate from 24 to 96 hours of incubation; use only approved fumigants as per manufacturer's directions

14

Poultry Wastes and Its Management

Pankaj Deka and Mihir Sarma

Poultry is one of the fastest-growing industries within agriculture and allied sectors worldwide. This rapid expansion results in the generation of substantial amounts of waste, including poultry manure, dead birds, hatchery wastes, and abattoir wastes. Proper treatment and scientific disposal of these wastes are crucial to avoid significant threats to both avian health and human safety. Unmanaged poultry wastes can lead to the spread of diseases among birds, resulting in considerable economic losses due to mortality and decreased productivity. Additionally, improper waste disposal can contribute to soil and groundwater pollution. Globally, an estimated 400 million chickens are processed weekly, generating a vast amount of waste. For instance, a broiler produces about 0.09 kg of manure daily, while a laying hen produces around 0.18 kg. Effective management of poultry waste requires a comprehensive understanding of its composition and the various physical, chemical, and microbiological processes that influence the fate of potential pollutants, particularly when the waste is applied to land.

Different types of poultry wastes and their management and disposal:

Table 14.1: Different poultry wastes with their disposal methods

Category	**Description**
	Types of Poultry Wastes
Poultry Manure	Composed of bedding materials, excreta, leftover feeds, feathers, etc.
Dead Birds	Birds that have died due to mortality.
Hatchery Wastes	Includes empty egg shells, infertile eggs, dead embryos, dead-in-germs, etc.
Slaughterhouse Wastes	Comprises feathers, blood, offals, and condemned carcasses from poultry processing.
	Management and Disposal
Solid Waste	Includes bedding material, excreta, feed remnants, feathers, hatchery waste, mortality waste.
Liquid Waste	Encompasses feces, urine, sawdust, remnants of drugs and pesticides, and wastewater from disinfection.
Techniques	Various methods for managing and disposing of poultry waste to reutilize nutrients and avoid risks.

Methods of disposal of poultry wastes

Disposing of poultry carcasses poses significant environmental, biological, and financial challenges for the poultry industry. Several methods are employed to manage these wastes effectively:

Table 14.2: List of methods of disposal of poultry wastes

Method	Description
Burial	- **Description**: Simple and cost-effective, especially for mass mortality due to diseases like Avian Influenza. - **Procedure**: Burial pit should be at least 91.44 meters away from wells, buildings, public roads, and utilities. Dead birds must be buried 0.91 to 2.44 meters deep. - **Concerns**: Risk of groundwater contamination and public perception issues if not properly sited.
Burning	- **Description**: Common among small-scale farmers, involves burning mortalities at high temperatures using fuels like wood, tires, or diesel. - **Concerns**: Can lead to atmospheric pollution, especially with outbreaks of highly infectious diseases. - **Site Requirements**: Must be located away from buildings, public roads, and utilities.
Incineration	- **Description**: A biologically safe method that destroys potentially infectious agents through thermal destruction. - **Concerns**: High costs, air pollution, and the need for careful control of emissions and residues. Not recommended for large-scale operations but beneficial for slaughter facilities.
Composting	- **Description**: Natural biological process that decomposes organic material into products that can be used as soil conditioners or fertilizers. - **Benefits**: Reduces poultry litter, stabilizes trace minerals, and reduces odors. Effective temperature range is between 40°C and 60°C. - **Concerns**: Loss of some nutrients, potential emission of greenhouse gases, and requires land area.
Rendering	- **Description**: Application of heat to remove fat from meat, producing products that can be used in animal feed, fertilizer, or further processed. - **Process**: Exposes materials to 133°C for at least 20 minutes at 3 bars. - **Uses**: Rendered products are used in animal feed, the chemical industry, or as fuel. - **Concerns**: Associated with gas and odor emissions.

Each disposal method has its advantages and challenges, and the choice of method should be based on factors such as scale of operation, environmental impact, and regulatory requirements.

A. **Management of poultry manure:** Poultry manure, a by-product of poultry farming, consists of feces, bedding materials, wasted feed, and feathers. As a substantial waste product from the poultry industry, it poses significant environmental challenges, including water, air, and land pollution. The high nitrogen content in poultry manure can lead to nitrate leaching, potentially contaminating groundwater and affecting drinking water sources. Proper management of poultry manure is crucial to mitigate these environmental impacts and harness its benefits. Effective strategies include drying to reduce moisture and pathogens, applying manure to soil to enhance fertility, and utilizing anaerobic digestion to produce biogas. Additionally, poultry manure can be repurposed as feed for cattle and fish, making it a valuable resource when managed appropriately.

Following is representation of the management practices for poultry wastes:

Table 14.3: Different poultry wastes, their composition and their utilities

Type of Waste	Description	Management Practices
Poultry Manure	Consists of feces, bedding materials, wasted feed, and feathers. Can lead to water, air, and land pollution.	- **Drying**: Economical method reducing moisture and destroying pathogens. - **Soil Application**: Direct spreading to improve soil fertility. - **Biogas Production**: Anaerobic digestion for energy recovery. - **Feed**: Used for cattle and fish, utilizing urea nitrogen.
Slaughterhouse Wastes	Includes feathers and skin, intestines, legs, and other by-products.	- **Rendering**: Produces meat-bone-meal for animal feed or fertilizer, and fat for various uses. - **Methane Production**: High methane yield from offal, blood, and bone meal. - **Preservation**: Use of formic acid to preserve by-products for feed.
Hatchery Wastes	Comprises egg shells, dead embryos, infertile eggs, and weak chicks.	- **Hatchery By-product Meal**: Conversion into protein-rich feed. - **Composting**: Kills pathogens and converts ammonia to organic nitrogen. - **Nutritional Value**: Dried dead embryos used in feed. - **Processing**: Boiling, soaking, sun-drying, or cooking and dehydrating for feed.

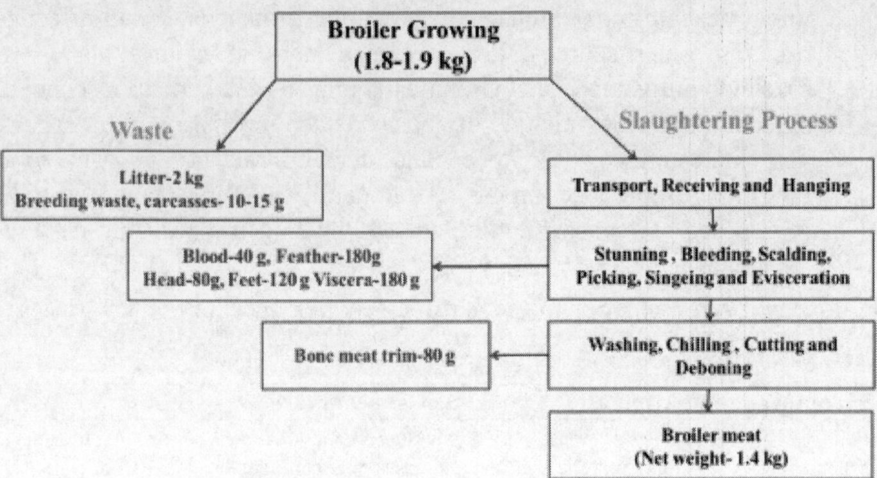

Fig. 14.1: Diagrammatic representation of broiler wastes

Source: Mozhiarasi and Natarajan, 2022

15

Management of Health Care, Medication and Bio-Security Measures

Pankaj Deka and Arfan Ali

Introduction

Poultry diseases pose a significant threat to commercial poultry production, often resulting in substantial economic losses due to high mortality and morbidity. Early diagnosis and effective management of these diseases are crucial, as many diseases share similar symptoms, making timely and accurate identification challenging. Poultry diseases can be broadly classified into bacterial, viral, fungal, protozoan, parasitic, and nutritional deficiency diseases. The following table provides an overview of these diseases, their causative agents, symptoms, and prevention and control measures.

Poultry Diseases Overview

Table 15.1: Different poultry diseases, their symptoms and prevention and control measures

Category	Disease	Causative Agent	Symptoms	Prevention and Control
Bacterial	**Pasteurellosis (Fowl Cholera)**	*Pasteurella multocida*	- **Per Acute:** High mortality with no visible signs - **Acute:** Depression, anorexia, mucus discharges, greenish diarrhea - **Chronic:** Depression, dyspnea, conjunctivitis, swollen wattles	- Medication - Vaccination - Rodent control
	Pullorum Disease	*Salmonella pullorum*	- Affects young chicks with high mortality - Depression, huddling, respiratory distress, weight loss, soiled vent, white chalky diarrhea, sudden death	- Slaughter of carriers - Routine serological testing of breeding stock - Hatchery hygiene - Rodent control

Category	Disease	Causative Agent	Symptoms	Prevention and Control
Viral	**Newcastle Disease (Ranikhet Disease)**	*Paramyxo virus type 1*	- **Acute:** Sudden death with no visible symptoms - **Sub Acute:** Depression, greenish diarrhea, cyanosis of comb, paralysis of wings, neck, legs, drop in egg production	- Vaccination
	Infectious Bursal Disease (Gumboro Disease)	*Birna virus*	- Depression, white watery diarrhea, soiled vent, anorexia, ruffled feathers, reluctance to move	- Vaccination
	Fowl Pox	*Fowl pox virus*	- Nodular proliferative skin lesions on non-feathered parts (head, neck, feet, legs) - Poor weight gain - Reduced egg production	- Vaccination - Mosquito control
	Marek's Disease	*Herpes virus*	- Depression before death - Transient paralysis - Enlargement of feather follicles - Tumors in organs like liver, gonad, skin, kidney, eye, bursa	- Vaccination
	Avian Influenza (Fowl Plague)	*Orthomyxovirus*	- **Low Pathogenic:** Respiratory signs (ocular and nasal discharge, sinusitis) - **High Pathogenic:** High mortality, cyanosis, edema of head, comb, wattle, blood-tinged discharges, greenish diarrhea, torticollis, incoordination	- Vaccination
Fungal	**Aspergillosis (Brooder Pneumonia)**	*Aspergillus fumigatus*	- Labored breathing - Gasping - Yellow to greenish nodules in lungs and air sacs	- Proper sanitation of hatchery, egg holding room, incubator, chick holding room - Dry litter management - Copper sulfate in drinking water

Category	Disease	Causative Agent	Symptoms	Prevention and Control
Protozoan	**Coccidiosis**	*Coccidial parasites*	- **Young Birds:** Bloody droppings, high mortality - **Adults:** Drop in feed consumption, egg production, emaciation	- Vaccination - Anticoccidial drugs - Proper hygiene and sanitation
Parasitic	**Ascariasis**	*Ascaridia galli*	- High parasitic load causing unthriftiness, poor growth, lower productivity	- Anthelmintics
	Caecal Worms	*Hetarakisgalli-nae*	- No obvious symptoms - Larvae can carry blackhead disease in turkeys	- Anthelmintics - Avoid rearing chickens with turkeys
	Ectoparasites	Mites, ticks, lice	- Irritation, blood-sucking, some act as vectors	- Good management and sanitation - Insecticides
Nutritional Deficiency	**Nutritional Roup**	Vitamin A deficiency	- Mucoid discharge from eyes and nasal passages - Decreased growth in chicks - Lowered egg production in layers	- Cod liver oil, fish oils, liver meal, green grasses
	Rickets	Vitamin D, calcium, phosphorus deficiency	- Lameness - Stiff legs - Swollen hocks - Rubbery beak - Drop in egg production	- Fish oils, sunlight, UV light, synthetic Vitamin D
	Nutritional Encephalomalacia (Crazy Chick Disease)	Vitamin E deficiency	- Incoordination - Convulsions - Paralysis of legs - Death	- Green grasses, vegetable oil, liver meal, legumes, synthetic Vitamin E
	Curled Toe Paralysis	Riboflavin (Vitamin B2) deficiency	- Poor growth - Paralysis of legs - Inward curling of toes- Tendency to walk on hocks	- Liver meal, milk by-products, young grasses, rice bran, molasses, synthetic Vitamin B2

General Measures for Prevention and Control of Poultry Diseases

Below is a tabular representation of the general measures for prevention and control of poultry diseases, including vaccination, deworming, treatment, litter management, and bio-security measures.

Table 15.2: Lists of general measures for prevention and control of poultry diseases

Measure	Details
Vaccination	**Precautions**: - Vaccinate only healthy flocks. - Use freshly stored vaccines, kept under refrigeration. - Vaccinate during cooler hours. - Follow sound management practices to minimize stress. - Keep accurate vaccine records.
Deworming	**Timing & Frequency**: - Start one week prior to Ranikhet disease vaccination (before 8 weeks of age). - Repeat every 3 weeks, totaling 4 dewormings before housing at 20 weeks.
Treatment	**Supervision**: - Ensure treatment is conducted as per a qualified veterinarian's instructions.
Litter Management	**Litter Conditions**: - Maintain optimal litter height. - Keep litter dry, turn frequently, and mix with lime.

Bio-Security Measures

Table 15.3: Different bio-security measures to be adopted in poultry farms

Measure	Details
Fencing & Visitor Control	- Secure farm with proper fencing. - Minimize visitors and limit visits to other poultry farms.
Wildlife Exclusion	- Prevent wild birds and animals from entering poultry houses.
Rodent & Pest Control	- Implement effective rodent and pest control programs.
Daily Inspections	- Inspect flocks daily to recognize disease symptoms early.
Ventilation & Cleanliness	- Ensure good ventilation and maintain dry litter. - Keep areas around houses and feed bins clean.
Equipment & Feed Control	- Avoid exchanging feed and equipment with other farms.
Disinfection & Sanitization	- Regularly disinfect poultry houses and equipment. - Use fumigation (formaldehyde & potassium permanganate) to sanitize poultry houses.
Foot Baths & Screening	- Install foot baths at the entrance of hatcheries and poultry sheds. - Conduct periodic screening of birds under veterinarian's guidance.

Guidelines for Proper Vaccination Program

Table 15.4: General guidelines for proper vaccination

Guideline	Details
Stress Management	- Use vaccines judiciously based on disease incidence in the farm and surrounding areas.
Vaccine Procurement & Storage	- Purchase vaccines from reliable sources. - Store vaccines under refrigeration (2° to 8°C) unless otherwise instructed.
Vaccination Schedule	- Follow the manufacturer's recommended schedule, including proper dosing and age.
Vaccine Expiry	- Never use expired or leftover vaccines.
Timing of Vaccination	- Vaccinate during cooler parts of the day, either early morning or late evening, especially in summer.
Health & Pre-Vaccination Care	- Vaccinate only healthy birds at their recommended ages. - Provide vitamins and anthelmintics at least a week before vaccination to reduce stress.
Water Vaccination Procedure	- When vaccinating through drinking water, keep birds thirsty for a few hours before administering the vaccine. - Use clean, cold drinking water free from chlorine or any other drugs for this purpose.

Table 15.5: Vaccination schedule for broiler chicken

Age	Name of the vaccine	Dose	Route
3 to 5th day	Ranikhet Disease (RD) Vaccine Lasota Strain	1 drop	Intraocular or intranasal
12 to 14th day	Infectious Bursal Disease (IBD)Vaccine Intermediate strain	1 drop	Intraocular or intranasal
16 to 18th day	Infectious Bursal Disease (IBD) Vaccine Intermediate strain (Booster)	-	Drinking water
24 to 26th day	Ranikhet Disease (RD) Vaccine Lasota Strain (Booster)	-	Drinking water

Table 15.6: Vaccination Schedule for commercial layer chicken:

Age	Name of the vaccine	Route
Day old	Marek's disease HVT- strain	Subcutaneous (S/C) at hatchery
5-7 days	Ranikhet disease Lasota strain	Nasal drop or Oral drop
14-15 days	Infectious Bursal disease(IBD)	Drinking water
4-5 weeks	Fowl pox 'BM' strain	Oral Drop or Drinking water
6-8 weeks	Ranikhet disease R_2B strain	Intramuscular (I/M)
8 weeks	Infectious Bursal disease (IBD) (Live) (Only in area of outbreak prone)	Intramuscular (I/M)
13-15 weeks	Infectious bronchitis	Oral Drop or Drinking water

14-15 weeks	Fowl pox ' BM' strain	Oral Drop or Drinking water
15-18 weeks	Egg drop Syndrome (Killed) Adjuvant	I/M
16-18 weeks	Ranikhet disease R_2B strain	I/M

Table 15.7: Vaccination schedule for duck

Disease	**Vaccine**	**Age of duck**	**Dose and route of administration**
Duck plague	Duck plague vaccine	6 weeks and above	0.5 ml S/C injection.
Duck cholera	Duck cholera vaccine	1st vaccine at 2-3 months 2nd vaccine after 1-2 months of 1st vaccination, then twice a year	0.5 ml S/C injection.

16

Organic and Hill Poultry Farming

Rafiqul Islam and Mustafizur Rahman

Organic Poultry Farming

Definition and Overview

- **The FAO/WHO Codex Alimentarius Commission** defines organic farming as a "holistic production management system that promotes and enhances agro-ecosystem health, including biodiversity, biological cycles, and soil biological activity, using non-farm agronomic, biological, and mechanical methods, excluding all synthetic off-farm inputs."
- **Organic chicken farming** involves raising chickens in a natural, humane environment outside of a conventional chicken house, feeding them organic feed (free from synthetic fertilizers, pesticides, and GMOs), and avoiding the use of antibiotics or growth hormones.
- The main goal is to produce healthier, environmentally friendly chicken products while ensuring high animal welfare standards.
- **Conversion Period**: Transitioning a conventional poultry farm to an organic one requires a certain period called the "conversion period."
- Organic poultry farming necessitates the use of **indigenous chicken varieties** managed organically, allowing the birds to express their natural behavior.
- **Growing Popularity**: The demand for organic poultry meat is increasing due to heightened health awareness among consumers. Chicken, in particular, has become a key organic meat due to its shorter production cycle.
- **Economic Consideration**: Organic poultry meat production is more cost-effective than organic livestock meat production, and India, with its vast population of indigenous chickens, has significant potential for organic poultry farming.

Advantages and Disadvantages of Organic Poultry Farming

Table 16.1: Lists of advantages and disadvantages of organic poultry farming

Advantages	Disadvantages
Sustainability: Promotes sustainable practices by efficiently utilizing natural resources and minimizing environmental impacts.	**Space Requirement**: Requires more space compared to commercial farming.
Reduced Chemical Use: Minimizes or eliminates the use of chemicals, reducing production costs and promoting healthier farming practices.	**Strict Regulations**: Farmers must adhere to strict rules, which may hinder successful transitions to organic production.
Waste Recycling: Encourages the recycling of organic waste, converting poultry waste into valuable fertilizers, supporting a closed-loop system.	**Consumer Awareness**: Limited consumer awareness about organic poultry farming leads to lower demand for organic eggs and meat.
Health Benefits: Organic chicken products are safer for human health, have better taste and nutritional profiles, and help reduce antibiotic-resistant bacteria.	**Higher Costs**: Organic eggs and meat are more expensive due to the stringent regulations governing organic poultry farming.
Animal Welfare: Emphasizes animal welfare by providing spacious housing with outdoor access, allowing chickens to exhibit natural behaviors.	**Infrastructure Challenges**: Lack of financial support, certification agencies, and marketing channels creates hurdles for organic poultry farming.
Market Value: Organic free-range chicken is a premium product, often sold at higher prices than conventional chicken, leading to potential higher profit margins.	**Long Conversion Period**: The transition from conventional to organic farming has a long conversion period, delaying full organic certification and benefits.
Support for Small Farmers: Organic chicken farming is suitable for small and marginal farmers, thereby supporting the local rural economy.	Higher Initial Costs: Setting up an organic poultry farm involves significant initial investment in infrastructure, organic feed, and certification processes, which can be a barrier for small-scale farmers.

Basic requirement for organic poultry production

Table 16.2: Basic requirements of organic poultry proudction

Basic Requirement	Details
1. Selection of Breed or Strain	• Local or indigenous breeds are preferred over exotic breeds due to better adaptation to local conditions and disease resistance. • Natural breeding techniques are favored, and parent stock must be purchased from organically certified sources.
2. Housing Management	• Organic housing should allow birds to express natural behaviors with minimal stress. • Adequate protection from predators, access to sunlight, shade, and open spaces are essential. • Deep litter system with clean, dry bedding (e.g., straw, wood shavings). • Minimum space requirements: 2 sq. ft per bird in confined space, 3 sq. ft per bird in foraging area. • Regular water quality testing, and proper ventilation.
3. Nutritional Management	• High-quality, organically grown feed provided. • Diet should allow natural eating habits. • Organic sources like peas, beans, rapeseed for protein. • Prebiotics, probiotics, and non-synthetic enzymes included. • Avoid synthetic amino acids; use organic substitutes. • Prevent excessive feeding.
4. Health Management	• Prevention prioritized with good sanitation and disinfection. • Avoid antibiotics; vaccinations permitted only when necessary. • Use of herbal remedies and natural additives for health improvement (e.g., Aloe vera, garlic, tulsi). • Growth promoters strictly forbidden.
5. Waste Management	• Easy disposal of excreta and manure with minimal soil and water degradation.
6. Transportation and Slaughter	• Transport with care to prevent stress, injury, and sickness. • Periodic water and food provision during transport. • Follow organic council guidelines for slaughter and packaging. • Separate rooms for slaughter processes, and chemical-free packaging.
7. Record Keeping	• Maintain detailed records for inspection by certifying organizations. • Types of records: Source of animal purchase, organic feed ingredients, feed supplements, treatment records, breeding details, pasture records, health care products, monthly flock records, egg packing/sales records, and other management records.
8. Conversion Period	• Simultaneous conversion of land and poultry recommended. • Minimum 12-month conversion phase for land before raising organic poultry. • Poultry must be raised for a specific period under organic management before products can be sold as organic. • Adherence to organic principles throughout the conversion process.

Hill poultry farming

Hill poultry farming is an agricultural practice that involves raising poultry in the hilly slopes or terrain of hills. This form of farming, also known as upland or terrace farming, is characterized by its adaptation to steep and challenging landscapes where traditional crop cultivation is difficult. Due to the rugged terrain, ploughing, planting, and harvesting crops can be arduous, and the soils are often prone to erosion and nutrient depletion. As a result, hill farming is better suited for livestock and poultry rearing. In recent years, hill poultry farming has gained traction, particularly in the north-eastern states of India, where it leverages the unique environmental conditions to raise poultry in a manner that complements the local geography and farming practices.

Table 16.3: Advantages and Disadvantages of Hill Poultry Farming

Advantages	**Disadvantages**
Efficient use of unused hilly terrains unsuitable for traditional agriculture.	Harsh climatic conditions, especially in winter, lead to high mortality among younger birds.
Scavenging feed resources such as pests, insects, and vegetative plants reduce feed costs.	Birds are more vulnerable to predators while scavenging.
Improves soil fertility.	Requires more space per bird compared to conventional poultry farming.
Suitable for organic meat and egg production, fetching a premium price.	Requires more manual labor.
Eggs produced have a yellowish yolk and special flavor, leading to higher demand in local markets.	Potential harm to local biodiversity of plants and animals.
	Farms are often not accessible by motorable roads, making transportation of inputs and outputs difficult.

Rearing Systems in Hill Poultry

Rearing System	**Description**
Free-Range System	Birds are let loose during the day and sheltered in an ordinary house made of locally available materials at night. Generally involves indigenous chickens that can escape predators.
Intensive System	Commercial chickens (broilers and layers) are kept inside sheds with proper ventilation, especially important at higher altitudes where oxygen concentration is low.

Management of Hill Poultry

Table 16.4: Lists of management of hill poultry

Aspect	Management Practices
Housing	In free-range systems, birds are housed at night in simple structures made from local materials. In intensive systems, sheds must be well-ventilated, and care should be taken to protect birds from chilling.
Feeding and Watering	Free-range birds scavenge for feed supplemented with kitchen waste. In intensive systems, balanced commercial feed is provided, with additional energy in winter to maintain body temperature.
Health Care	Proper brooding, ventilation, and prevention of wet litter are essential to avoid cold shock, suffocation, and high ammonia levels. Respiratory diseases are more common in high altitudes, requiring special care.
Incubation and Hatching	Lower oxygen levels at high altitudes can reduce hatchability, so commercial hatcheries should be located at lower altitudes for optimal results.

17

Poultry Based Mixed and Integrated Farming

Mihir Sarma and Rafiqul Islam

Mixed and Integrated Poultry Farming

Mixed farming refers to the practice of cultivating crops and rearing livestock on the same farm, aimed at maximizing economic benefits through the efficient use of resources. This type of farming can be practiced either simultaneously or at different times, depending on the needs and conditions. In India, mixed farming is particularly significant as it typically contributes at least 10% of a farmer's income from livestock, potentially reaching up to 49%.

Advantages of Mixed Farming

- **Maximized Returns:** By-products of farm activities, such as crop residues, can be effectively utilized to feed livestock, leading to higher returns.
- **Year-Round Employment:** Mixed farming provides continuous work opportunities throughout the year, ensuring a steady income.
- **Efficient Resource Utilization:** The combination of crops and livestock ensures optimal use of land, labor, and capital.
- **Soil Fertility:** Livestock manure contributes to maintaining and enhancing soil fertility, which is crucial for sustained crop production.
- **Balanced Food Production:** Mixed farming allows for the production of a variety of food items, leading to a more balanced diet throughout the year.
- **Increased Social Status:** The diverse activities involved in mixed farming can enhance the social status of farmers by increasing their income and self-sufficiency.
- **Risk Reduction:** Mixed farming reduces dependency on external inputs and mitigates risks associated with natural calamities by diversifying income sources.

- **Environmental Sustainability:** It is an eco-friendly approach that supports the efficient recycling of nutrients and resources within the farm system.
- **Self-Reliance:** Mixed farming fosters a general level of self-reliance within the farming community, reducing the need for external inputs.

Examples of Mixed Farming Systems

i) **Duck-cum-Fish Farming:** This system is highly common and involves the rearing of ducks alongside fish farming. Ducks act as natural manuring agents for the ponds, aerating the water and controlling pests like frogs and dragonflies. A typical setup might involve 300 ducks per hectare of water spread area, effectively fertilizing the pond and contributing to fish production.

ii) **Duck-Pig-Fish-Vegetable Farming System:** Widely practiced in Southeast Asia and China, this system integrates pond-based farming with pigs, ducks, and fish, alongside vegetable production. The pond water is utilized to meet the needs of pigs and ducks, while also supporting fish farming and vegetable cultivation.

iii) **Poultry-cum-Fish Farming:** An economically viable system, poultry-cum-fish farming can yield fish production levels of 4500-5000 kg per hectare. Poultry droppings serve as direct feed for fish species like common carp, enhancing water productivity. One adult chicken produces about 25 to 30 kg of manure in one year. In the poultry-cum-fish farming system, this manure can be effectively utilized to fertilize fish ponds, enhancing the biological productivity of the water. Typically, 500-600 chickens are sufficient to fertilize one hectare of pond area. This integration not only provides a sustainable source of nutrients for fish farming but also ensures that the by-products of poultry farming are fully utilized, contributing to the overall efficiency and profitability of the mixed farming system. Deep litter poultry manure is applied daily at a rate of 40-50 kg/hectare, depending on the water quality.

iv) **Poultry-cum-Pig-cum-Fish Farming:** This is one of the most profitable mixed farming systems. It involves the integration of poultry, pigs, and fish farming, where 270 chickens are kept alongside 30 pigs. The excreta from the pigs are sufficient to fertilize a one-hectare pond area for fish farming. This system is highly efficient and productive, making it an attractive option for farmers seeking to maximize their income.

v) **Rice-Duck Mixed Farming:** In this system, ducks are raised alongside rice cultivation. Ducks help control pests and weeds in the rice fields, reducing the need for chemical pesticides and manual weeding. Additionally, their droppings act as natural fertilizer for the rice crops, minimizing the use of chemical fertilizers.

Integrated Mixed Farming

Agriculture remains a major employment sector in India, particularly for small and marginal farmers and agricultural laborers. However, these groups often face challenges such as unemployment or underemployment due to the seasonal nature of crop production and natural calamities. Integrated mixed farming offers a solution by providing regular employment opportunities through the combination of various farming enterprises.

Advantages of Integrated Mixed Farming

- **Higher Employment Potential:** Integrated farming systems offer more employment opportunities than single enterprise farming by involving multiple activities such as livestock rearing, crop production, and aquaculture.
- **Sustainable Development:** Integrating different components like poultry, pigs, ducks, and fish ensures better utilization of land, water, and other resources, contributing to the overall sustainability of the farming model.
- **Economic Viability:** The integrated model is economically viable and helps uplift the rural economy by providing multiple streams of income to farmers.
- **Resource Efficiency:** Integrated farming promotes the efficient use of inputs and outputs, reducing waste and improving productivity.
- **Risk Management:** By diversifying income sources, integrated farming reduces the risks associated with market fluctuations and environmental changes, providing greater financial stability to farmers.

Integrated Farming System (IFS)

The Integrated Farming System (IFS) involves the integration of various farm enterprises-such as crops, livestock, aquaculture, poultry, sericulture, and agro-forestry-to achieve economic and sustainable agricultural production through the efficient utilization of resources. The key principle of IFS is that waste generated from one component serves as an input for another, promoting efficient recycling within the system. FAO (2017) stated that 'there is no waste', and 'waste is only a misplaced resource which can become a valuable material for another product' in IFS.

Key Components of Integrated Farming System (IFS)

1. **Agriculture (Field Crops):** Cultivation of various crops such as grains, legumes, and vegetables. It forms the base of the farming system and provides food, feed, and raw materials for other components.
2. **Horticulture:** Involves the cultivation of fruits, vegetables, and ornamental plants. It adds diversity to the farming system and provides additional sources of nutrition and income.
3. **Agro-forestry:** The integration of trees and shrubs with crops and livestock. It enhances biodiversity, improves soil fertility, and provides timber, fuel, and fodder.
4. **Mushroom Cultivation:** Cultivating edible fungi such as mushrooms. It utilizes organic waste products and provides a high-protein food source.
5. **Sericulture:** The production of silk through the rearing of silkworms. It offers an additional income source and uses mulberry leaves grown in the system.
6. **Poultry:** Rearing of chickens, ducks, or turkeys for meat and eggs. Poultry provides a source of protein and its waste products can be used as fertilizer.
7. **Pigeon Rearing:** Raising pigeons for meat (squab) and as pets. It complements other components by utilizing waste and providing a secondary source of income.
8. **Rabbitry:** Rearing rabbits for meat and fur. Rabbits are efficient converters of feed into meat and their manure can be used as a high-quality fertilizer.
9. **Duck Rearing:** Raising ducks for meat and eggs. Ducks can help in pest control and their waste can be used to fertilize aquatic systems.
10. **Azolla Farming:** Cultivation of Azolla, a type of water fern used as green manure or livestock feed. It fixes nitrogen and improves soil fertility.
11. **Fodder Production:** Growing plants specifically for animal feed. Fodder crops are essential for maintaining livestock health and productivity.
12. **Vermiculture:** The cultivation of earthworms for producing vermicompost. This process converts organic waste into high-quality fertilizer.
13. **Piggery:** Rearing pigs for meat. Pigs can utilize various waste products and their manure is valuable for fertilizing crops.

14. **Seed Production:** Growing crops specifically for seed production. It ensures the availability of quality seeds for future planting.
15. **Sheep Rearing:** Raising sheep for meat (lamb or mutton), wool, and milk. Sheep contribute to the system by providing various products and utilizing crop residues.
16. **Goat Rearing:** Rearing goats for meat (chevon), milk, and fiber. Goats are versatile and can thrive on a variety of feed sources.
17. **Dairy:** The production of milk from cattle, buffaloes, or goats. Dairy farming provides essential nutrients and generates income.
18. **Apiary:** Beekeeping for honey and other bee products. Bees also contribute to pollination, which enhances crop yields.
19. **Aquaculture:** The farming of fish, shellfish, and other aquatic organisms. It provides a protein-rich food source and can be integrated with other farming activities.

Each component of the IFS works synergistically to enhance productivity, sustainability, and economic viability, leveraging the strengths and waste products of each enterprise.

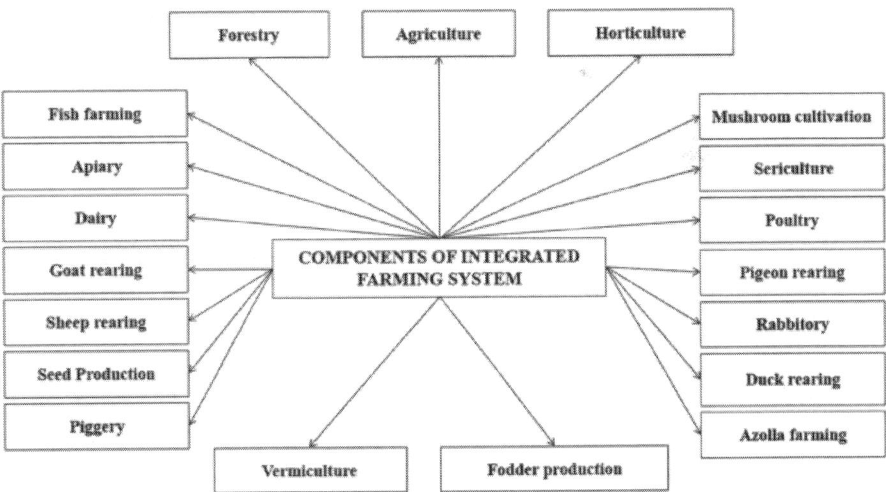

Fig.17.1: Different components of integrated farming system

Source: Bhagat et al., 2024

Table 17.2: Advantages of Integrated Farming System

Advantage	Description
Productivity	Increases economic yield per unit area per unit time by intensifying crop and allied enterprises.
Profitability	Reduces production costs through effective use of waste material and byproducts, improving profitability and benefit-cost ratio.
Sustainability	Organic inputs from one subsystem sustain the production base for longer periods compared to monoculture systems.
Balanced Food	Provides diverse sources of nutrition by integrating different food sources, meeting all nutrient requirements.
Environmental Safety	Minimizes environmental pollution through effective recycling of waste materials.
Recycling	Cornerstone of IFS, recycling products, byproducts, and waste materials effectively, especially in resource-poor rural areas.
Income Round the Year	Ensures a continuous flow of income through interactions of various enterprises (crops, eggs, meat, milk).
Saving Energy	Reduces dependency on fossil fuels by using cattle for transportation and cow dung for cooking or biogas.
Meeting Fodder Crisis	Utilizes crop residues as fodder for livestock and grains as feed for monogastric animals, addressing fodder shortages.
Employment Generation	Creates job opportunities by combining crop and livestock enterprises, increasing labor requirements and reducing underemployment.

Different Poultry-Based Integrated Farming Models

Table 17.3: Different types of poultry-based integrated farming system

Sl. No.	Model	Description
a	Crop + Dairy + Fish + Poultry	Integration of crops, dairy, fish, and poultry to utilize resources efficiently.
b	Crop + Dairy + Poultry + Vermicompost	Combines crop, dairy, poultry, and vermicomposting to recycle waste and improve soil fertility.
c	Fruit Crops + Fishery + Poultry	Integrates fruit cultivation, fish farming, and poultry to diversify production and utilize waste.
d	Crop + Horticulture + Dairy + Sheep + Poultry	Combines multiple enterprises to optimize resource use and increase farm productivity.
e	Crops + Horticulture + Cattle + Fishery + Poultry + Apiary	A comprehensive model incorporating various enterprises for maximum resource utilization and productivity.
f	Crop + Dairy + Fishery Cum Duckery	Integrates crop cultivation, dairy, fishery, and duck farming for effective resource use and production.

Sl. No.	Model	Description
g	Field Crop + Fish + Duck + Goat	Combines field crops, fish, ducks, and goats to optimize resource utilization and production.
h	Crop + Fish + Poultry	A simple model integrating crops, fish, and poultry for efficient use of resources and space.
i	Poultry-Fish Culture	Integrates poultry with fish culture to reduce costs and maximize benefits by using poultry excreta to fertilize fish ponds.
j	Poultry Raising for Meat (Broilers) or Eggs (Layers) with Fish Culture	Poultry and fish culture integration to cut fertilizer costs and utilize space effectively.
k	Poultry Dung Utilization	Poultry dung used as fertilizer for fish ponds, reducing fish production costs by 60%. 25-30 birds can produce 1 tonne of dip litter annually.
l	Duck-Fish Culture	Ducks and fish are integrated to enhance fish production, reduce costs, and improve pond health. Ducks act as living manure machines and help in controlling pests.
m	Advantages of Duck-Fish Integration	Increases fish production, reduces fish culture costs, and enhances pond health. Ducks provide nutrients and control pests in the pond.

Table 17.4: Limitations of Livestock-Based Integrated Farming System

Limitation	Description
Digestibility of Crop Residues	Lower digestibility and protein content of crop residues lead to reduced nutritional benefits; treatments are expensive or unavailable for small farmers.
Neglect of Crop Residues	Often neglected or misapplied despite their role in regenerating soil.
Nutrient Losses	Intensive recycling can result in nutrient losses.
Cost of Manure Fertilizer	Higher production and transportation costs if manure use efficiency is not improved.
Preference for Chemical Fertilizers	Chemical fertilizers are preferred for their ease of use over manure.
Manure Transportation	Increased investments needed for manure use and transportation, especially in mixed farms.

Opportunities of Livestock-Based Integrated Farming System

Table 17.5: List of opportunities of livestock based integrated farming system

Opportunity	**Description**
Intensification of Agriculture	Favorable conditions for integrating livestock as agriculture intensifies.
Fertilizer and Labor Shortages	Reliance on manure due to high fertilizer prices and labor shortages.
Seasonal Livestock Enterprise	Opportunities for livestock enterprises during the dry season while growing crops in the wet season.
Economic Advantage of Livestock	Livestock enterprises are often more profitable than crop farming, making integration advantageous.
Technological Support	Availability of technologies to support sustainable crop-livestock integration.

The Integrated Farming System (IFS) offers a viable solution for small and marginal farmers by enhancing nutritional and economic status, creating employment opportunities, and optimizing resource use. Proper documentation and dissemination of various IFS models are crucial for improving the livelihoods of rural and urban populations.

18

Integration in Commercial Poultry Production: Contract Farming

Mustafizur Rahman and Ashim Kumar Saikia

Integrated Poultry Farming

Integration refers to the coordination and amalgamation of various stages in poultry production to create a seamless flow of inputs and outputs, reducing overall production costs. This approach ensures that each stage of production, from breeding to marketing, is efficiently managed within a unified system.

- **Global Integration:** In developed countries, poultry production is highly integrated, encompassing all stages from principal breeding to consumer distribution. This includes broiler farms, hatcheries, feed mills, processing plants, and animal healthcare products, which work together to streamline production and marketing processes.
- **Indian Context:** In India, integration and contract farming in poultry began with Suguna Poultry Farm Limited in 1991. While this marked the start of integration in broiler production, it did not fully represent the comprehensive integration seen in more developed systems.
- **Current Practice in India:** Integrators provide essential inputs such as chicks, feed, medicines, vaccines, and technical support. They also handle marketing of the final product. Poultry farmers, operating as contract growers, receive payments based on the weight of broilers or number of eggs produced. Despite these developments, integration within the layer sector remains underdeveloped in India.

Integration in poultry farming aims to improve efficiency, reduce costs, and ensure better quality control through a coordinated approach across all production stages.

Different types of integration

Table 18.1: Different types integrations used in commercial poultry farming

Type of Integration	Description	Function	Advantages
Vertical Integration	Linking different stages of poultry production (breeding, hatchery, farming, processing, marketing) within a single firm.	Outputs from one stage become inputs for the next, reducing transaction costs and improving quality control.	Reduces overall production costs, minimizes transaction costs, enhances supply chain control, and lowers final product costs.
Horizontal Integration	Merging units involved in the same stage of production (e.g., multiple breeding farms or hatcheries).	Increases operational scale and efficiency, and may involve co-operative buying groups.	Enhances production capacity, achieves economies of scale, and reduces unit costs.
Parallel Integration	Diversifying into related industries (e.g., a hatchery operator starts manufacturing incubators).	Reduces core business production costs and generates additional revenue.	Creates new income streams, lowers production costs, and provides control over related products.
Forward Integration	Gaining control over downstream business activities (e.g., selling directly to customers).	Skips intermediaries to improve control over distribution and customer experience.	Reduces dependency on intermediaries, enhances market presence, and improves customer control.
Backward Integration	Gaining control over upstream business activities (e.g., securing raw material supply).	Manages and controls sources of raw materials and inputs.	Ensures reliable supply, reduces input costs, and enhances quality and availability control.

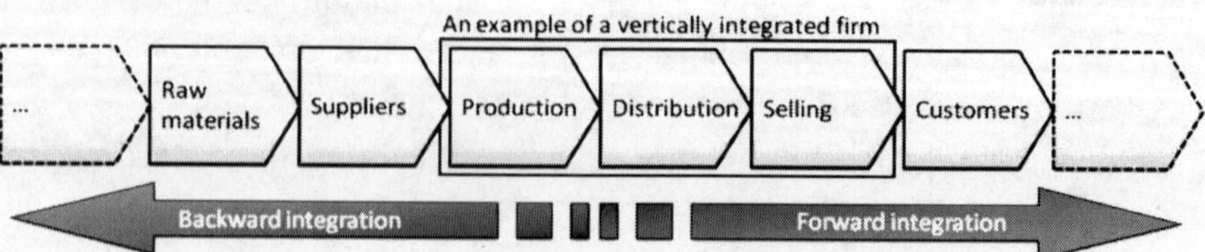

Fig. 18.1: The concept of vertical integration (adapted from Porter, 1980)

Advantages and disadvantages of integration

Table 18.2: List of advantages in integration in commercial poultry farming

Advantages	Description
Reduces marketing expenses	Integration streamlines the supply chain, reducing costs associated with marketing and distribution.
Certainty of supplies of materials and services	Ensures a stable and reliable supply of inputs, minimizing disruptions and uncertainties.
Better control over product distribution	Allows for direct management of distribution channels, improving efficiency and reach.
Tighter quality control of the final product	Facilitates comprehensive monitoring and quality assurance throughout the production process.
Additional profit margins or the ability to charge lower prices on final products	Reduces costs and enhances profitability, or allows for more competitive pricing.
Better inventory control	Improves management of stock levels, reducing waste and shortages.

Table 18.3: List of disadvantages in integration in commercial poultry farming

Disadvantages	Description
Higher capital investment	Requires significant upfront investment to integrate various stages of production.
Threats to smaller individual farmers	Can marginalize smaller farmers, making it difficult for them to compete.
Integration often results in regional monopolies	Can lead to market dominance by a few large players, reducing competition.
Potential to lose the national, regional, or individual identity of an organization	May lead to a loss of unique characteristics and local relevance.
Loss of independence for decision making	Can reduce the autonomy of individual farmers or smaller firms within the integrated system.

Contract Farming in Poultry Production

Contract farming is an agreement between farmers and processing or marketing firms for the production and supply of agricultural products. These agreements often involve predetermined prices and are designed to streamline the production and supply chain.

Key Aspects

- The term ‘contract’ in broiler production can vary by country and the specific integration company.
- Contracts specify the conditions for producing and marketing broilers between farmers (growers) and integrators (contractors).

- Contract farming in broiler production began before 1960 in many developed countries and was introduced in India in 1991 by Suguna Poultry Farm Limited (now Suguna Foods).
- Vertically integrated contract farming is widely adopted globally.

Roles and Responsibilities

- **Integrators/Contractors:** Provide day-old chicks, feed, medication, technical support, and transportation.
- **Farmers/Growers:** Provide land, housing facilities, labor, and cover other operational expenses such as repairs, maintenance, manure disposal, and poultry house cleaning.

Benefits

- Provides technology, extension services, financial credit, and an assured market for farmers.
- Helps in overcoming credit constraints and minimizing transaction costs.

Challenges

- Contract farming may lead to unequal partnerships, with farmers being the weaker party and potentially vulnerable to exploitation by integrators.

Payment Structure

1. **Base Payment:** A fixed charge per kg of live broiler.
2. **Incentive or Performance Payment:** A percentage of the difference between average settlement costs for all flocks during a specific period and the cost associated with the individual grower.
3. **Disaster Payment:** Terms for compensation in case of unforeseen issues affecting production.

This system helps in streamlining production and marketing but also poses challenges related to fairness and balance in the contractual relationship.

Advantages of Contract Farming

Table 18.4: List of advantages of contract farming

Advantage	Description
Overcoming Credit Constraints	Vertically integrated contract farming helps overcome credit constraints and provides financial support.
Minimizing Transaction Costs	Reduces transaction costs through direct relationships between farmers and integrators.
Unification of Small Farmers	Integrates low-income small farmers into the commercial poultry sector, providing them with opportunities.
Reduced Production Costs	Minimizes costs due to reduced involvement of middlemen and streamlined processes.
Quality Assurance	Ensures high-quality poultry production, with methods proven effective worldwide.
Guaranteed Minimum Price	Provides a guaranteed minimum price for farmers, protecting them from price volatility.
Simplified Farming Role	Simplifies the farmer's role, making it accessible to uneducated and under-employed individuals in rural areas.
Lower Production Costs	Production costs are typically 20% lower compared to independent farming due to efficiencies in the system.
Marketing Managed by Integrators	Farmers are relieved from marketing concerns, as integrators handle the marketing of the broilers.

Disadvantages of Contract Farming

Table 18.5: List of disadvantages of contract farming

Disadvantage	Description
Favoritism Towards Larger Growers	Larger growers may benefit more, potentially leaving smaller or poorer growers behind.
Threats to Small-Scale Farmers	Small-scale poultry farmers may face challenges and risks under the contract farming system.
Loss of Decision-Making Independence	Farmers may lose control over key decisions related to their production and operations.
Potential for Agreement Manipulation	Contractors might exploit or manipulate contract terms to their advantage, potentially disadvantaging farmers.

19

Other Avian Species and Their Management

Rafiqul Islam

Management of Other Avian Species

Duck

Overview

- **Asia:** The homeland of ducks.
- **Global Rankings:** China holds the first position in duck population, followed by India.
- **Significance in India:** Ducks are the second most important poultry species, constituting about 10% of the total poultry population (851.82 million) and contributing 6-7% of the total egg production (138.38 billion) in the country (BAHS, 2024).

Regional Distribution

- **Leading States:** West Bengal leads in duck population, followed by Assam, Bihar, Manipur, Kerala, Andhra Pradesh, Tamil Nadu, Orissa, Tripura, and Jammu & Kashmir.
- **Consumption:** Major consumers of duck eggs and meat include West Bengal, Assam, and Kerala.

Advantages of Duck Farming

Table 19.1: Common advantages of duck farming

Advantage	**Description**
Efficient Feed Conversion	Ducks can convert low-quality waste materials into high-quality protein.
Minimal Housing Requirements	Ducks require simple housing and less care compared to chickens.
Prolific Egg Layers	Native breeds can lay 160-180 eggs annually under extensive rearing systems.
Larger Egg Size	Duck eggs are 10-15% larger than chicken eggs.
Natural Pest Control	Ducks help exterminate harmful insects in crop fields, increasing crop production and reducing feed costs.
Hardiness and Disease Resistance	Ducks are hardy, more easily brooded, and resistant to many avian diseases.
No Cannibalism	Ducks are free from cannibalism and other objectionable tendencies.
Integration with Crop and Fish Culture	Duck farming can be easily integrated with crop and fish culture, reducing feed costs and increasing profit margins.

Duck Breeds

Table 19.2: Common breeds of duck

Category	**Breed**	**Description**
Domesticated Breeds	Most domesticated ducks are descendants of the wild mallard. Many indigenous ducks in India are of nondescript types.	
Registered Native Breeds	Pati, Maithili, Andamani	These are Indian native breeds registered under ICAR-NBAGR, Karnal.
Meat-Type Breeds	Pekin, Aylesbury, Muscovy, Rouen, Cayuga, Buff, Swedish	Breeds used primarily for meat production.
Egg-Type Breeds	Indian Runner, Khaki Campbell	Breeds known for high egg production.
Ornamental Breeds	Call, Crested White, Black East India	Breeds kept for ornamental purposes.

Extensive or nomadic system of duck rearing

The extensive or nomadic system of duck rearing is the most prevalent method of duck farming in India, particularly among landless agricultural laborers who rely on it as their primary source of income. This traditional system involves minimal scientific intervention, with ducks allowed to forage freely in harvested paddy fields or waterways, and housed in basic bamboo enclosures at night. Financial assistance for these farmers often comes from landlords or egg vendors, with repayments made through eggs or spent birds. The entire process, from hatching to laying, is closely tied to the agricultural cycle, with hatching synchronized with rice harvesting seasons. Despite the challenges of seasonal feeding and migration in search of resources, this system remains integral to rural livelihoods, with ducks playing a vital role in controlling insect populations and maximizing feed efficiency. The following table outlines the key aspects of this rearing method.

Table 19.3: Some key aspects of nomadic system of duck rearing

Aspect	Details
Commonality	Most common system of duck rearing in India.
Primary Farmers	Agricultural landless labor group, relying solely on duck farming for income.
Housing and Feeding	Scientific housing and feeding systems are generally not practiced.
Financial Assistance	Farmers often obtain financial aid from landlords or egg vendors, repaid typically in eggs or spent birds.
Flock Size	Expressed in dozens, averaging 15 dozen with a range of 10-25 dozen ducks.
Foraging	Ducks forage in harvested paddy fields or waterways; held in bamboo enclosures or raised houses at night.
Lean Season Feeding	Ducks are hand-fed with grains like paddy and sorghum, and sometimes unsalted fish or palm pith.
Egg Collection and Sale	Eggs collected cleanly for hatching and sold at 8-10% higher prices than chicken eggs.
Egg Handling	Wholesale vendors often candle eggs before transportation.
Hatching Season	Synchronized with rice harvesting, occurring in October-November and January-February.
Hatching Method	Broody hens are used, with about 20 eggs per hen; incubation lasts 28 days.
Hatchability	Typically above 60%, with experienced farmers achieving 80-85%.
Duckling Management	Ducklings removed from broody hen on the second day, confined in temporary sheds for 7 days, then hand-fed with broken rice grains and rice bran.
Foraging After 7-10 Days	Ducklings are allowed on waterways, and after one month, they forage on harvested paddy fields and wet areas.
Laying Age	Ducks start laying at about 6 months of age.
Flock Management	Farmers maintain flocks for two years of production or purchase layer ducks for another year.
Surplus Ducks	Surplus drakes and spent ducks are sold for meat.
Challenges	Migration in search of fresh feeding resources, hand-feeding during lean seasons, and in-between harvests leads to losses.

Aspect	Details
Benefits in Developing Countries	Ducks act as scavengers, utilizing insects and improving feed efficiency while reducing insect problems.
Special Practices in China	Ducks are trained to ingest grasshoppers, protecting agricultural lands from damage.

Semi-intensive or intensive system of duck rearing

The semi-intensive and intensive systems of duck rearing have gained popularity as alternatives to the traditional free-range method, which, while cost-effective in terms of feed, requires extensive land. These systems offer more controlled environments that optimize space and resources. In the semi-intensive system, ducklings are provided with a combination of covered areas and running space, with wire-net fencing and concrete water channels to maintain hygiene and facilitate feeding. The intensive system, on the other hand, can involve either floor housing or cage housing, with an emphasis on maintaining cleanliness through the use of wire-floored houses. Despite being waterfowl, ducks do not require swimming water at any stage of rearing, making these systems more adaptable to different environments.

The features of the semi-intensive and intensive systems:

Table 19.4: Some key aspects of semi-intensive system of duck rearing

System	Key Features
Semi-Intensive	- 135 m² covered area per duckling
	- 1.35-1.80 m² running space per duckling
	- Wire-net fencing (60 cm high)
	- Watering and feeding arrangements in the run
	- Concrete water channel (60 cm wide, 30 cm deep) alongside rearing houses
	- Laying nests (30 x 30 x 45 cm) provided for every 3 ducks
Intensive	- Floor housing (deep-litter or wire-floored)
	- Cage housing
	- Wire-floored houses preferred for hygiene
	- No need for swimming water

Geese

Geese, belonging to the Anseriformes Anatidae family, are waterfowls known for their excellent foraging abilities. In India, the brown-backed and white geese are commonly found, with "Kashmir Anz" being the first recognized breed in the country. These birds are hardy and can adapt to various feeding and management conditions, making them a viable option for farming. Geese reach sexual maturity at around two years and can lay between 30 to 50 eggs annually. They are also known for their longevity, with a life span of 10-20 years. Below is a table summarizing the key aspects of geese farming:

Table 19.5: Some key features of geese

Aspect	Details
Species	Geese (Anseriformes Anatidae)
Common Breeds	Brown-backed, White Geese, Kashmir Anz (first recognized breed in India)
Body Weights	Gander: 3.82 kg, Goose: 3.34 kg (Kashmir Anz breed)
Sound	Honking
Sexual Maturity	Around 2 years
Egg Production	30 to 50 eggs annually (varies with breed, nutrition)
Egg Weight	144 to 150 g
Life Span	10-20 years
Advantages	- Hardy and adaptable to different conditions - Can digest 40-50% crude fibre - Fastest growing poultry species - High feed conversion efficiency (FCE)

Housing

Geese are generally not reared in total confinement, which allows them to take advantage of their natural foraging instincts. The most common housing system for geese is the semi-intensive system, which provides a balance between shelter and freedom to forage.

Semi-Intensive Housing System for Geese

Table 19.6: Some important aspects of geese rearing

Aspect	Description
Shelter and Night Housing	Basic shelter with adequate ventilation and protection from weather; spacious with dry bedding material.
Foraging During the Day	Geese are let loose to graze on pasturelands during the day, reducing feed costs and providing exercise.
Pasture Management	One hectare of pasture supports 50-100 geese; rotational grazing to prevent overgrazing and allow recovery.
Water Access	Clean water for drinking and occasional bathing; water containers placed in shaded areas.
Fencing	Fenced foraging area to contain geese and protect from predators; typically around 1 meter in height.
Feed and Water Stations	Supplementary feeding during lean seasons; feed and water stations located in shaded areas or within shelter.

By combining adequate shelter with ample opportunities for natural foraging, the semi-intensive system ensures that geese are healthy, productive, and able to express their natural behaviors, leading to more sustainable and profitable farming.

Table 19.7: Floor, feeder and drinker space requirement of duck and geese:

Age	**Duck**	**Geese**
Floor space (m^2/bird)		
Brooder (Hover) space	0.003	0.0035
0-4 weeks	0.072	0.135
4-8 weeks	0.135	0.180
8-12 weeks	0.180	0.270
>12 weeks	0.270	0.450
Adult	0.450-0.540	0.720
Feeder space (cm/bird)		
0-1 week	5.0	5.0
1-2 weeks	5.0	6.25
2-4 weeks	6.25	7.5
4-8 weeks	6.25	10.0
>8 weeks	7.5	12.5
Adult	12.5	15.0
Drinker space (cm/bird)		
0-1 week	1.75	1.75
1-4 weeks	1.75	2.5
4-8 weeks	1.75	2.5
>8 weeks	2.0	3.0
Adult	2.5	3.5
		Source: Wilson *et. al.*, 1997

Feeding

Feeding geese involves catering to their primarily herbivorous diet, which includes a variety of natural foods such as shoots, seeds, stems, roots, grass, berries, bulbs, and grains. Geese are efficient grazers and can largely acquire their feed through foraging. Goslings, the young geese, predominantly eat grass. For drinking, it is essential to provide wide and deep drinkers (either pans or troughs) that allow the geese to dip both their bill and head. For scientific feeding practices, geese are also known to prefer pellets, and their diet should be balanced to meet specific nutritional requirements for optimal growth and health.

Table 19.8: Nutrient requirement of geese:

Nutrients	0-2 weeks	3-7 weeks	Breeder
Metabolizable Energy, kcal/kg	2900	3000	2900
Crude Protein, %	20	15	15
Lysine, %	1.0	0.85	0.60
Methionine + Cystine, %	0.6	0.5	0.5
Calcium, %	0.65	0.6	2.25
Phosphorus, non-phytin, %	0.30	0.30	0.30
Vitamin A, IU/kg	1500	4000	4000
Vitamin D3, ICU/kg	200	200	200
Riboflavin, mg/kg	3.8	2.5	4.0

Other management

In managing geese, several key practices ensure successful rearing and production. Goslings can be brooded artificially but should be introduced to short grass as soon as possible to benefit from natural foraging. Maintaining a proper breeding ratio and providing adequate nesting arrangements are crucial for effective reproduction. Natural incubation is preferred, with a period of 29-31 days, although Egyptian geese may require up to 35 days. To enhance hatchability, eggs should be moistened and manually turned if necessary. Prompt removal of hatched goslings to a warm environment is important to prevent the brooding goose from neglecting unhatched eggs.

Geese are valuable for their foraging abilities, which can help control weeds in crop fields. They are relatively resilient to diseases but can be affected by internal parasites, necessitating regular deworming. The following table summarizes these management practices for efficient and productive geese farming.

Table 19.9: Some key management aspects of geese

Aspect	Details
Brooding and Release	Goslings can be brooded artificially; release onto short grass as soon after hatching as possible.
Litter Management	Manage litter carefully due to high moisture content in faecal materials to avoid wet litter problems.
Breeding Ratio	Maintain a ratio of 5 geese per gander for effective breeding.
Breeding Observations	Monitor gender to avoid preferential mating during the breeding season.
Nesting	Provide one nest for every three geese to ensure clean eggs and avoid soiled or floor eggs.
Incubation	Typically natural incubation under chickens, ducks, or turkeys with 29-31 days period (35 days for Egyptian geese). Use water sprinkling or dipping to enhance hatchability. Manual turning needed if using chickens.

Aspect	Details
Weeding and Feeding	Geese can clear unwanted plants from crops. Goslings aged 6 weeks should be fed light grain feed at night and released in fields the next morning.
Health Management	Regular deworming is essential to control internal parasites, as geese may pick up worm eggs while foraging.

Japanese Quail (*Coturnix coturnix japonica*)

The Japanese quail (*Coturnix coturnix japonica*) is a small, agile bird renowned for its rapid growth and prolific egg production. Native to Asia, these quails are particularly valued in India for both their meat and eggs. They are well-suited to a variety of environments and do not require complex housing or extensive space, making them an attractive option for small-scale and backyard farming. Their quick maturity, high egg yield, and adaptability have established them as a favored species among poultry enthusiasts and commercial producers alike.

Table 19.10: Some special features and advantages of quail farming:

Feature	Details
Size and Weight	**Male Quail:** 120-150 g **Female Quail:** 150-180 g
Age at Marketing	5-6 weeks
Market Weight	Approximately 250 g at 5-6 weeks of age
Age at Sexual Maturity	6-7 weeks
Annual Egg Production	About 280 eggs per bird
Incubation Period	17-18 days
Average Egg Weight	10 g
Nutritional Benefits of Meat	Lower fat content compared to chicken meat; beneficial for body and brain development, suitable for children, patients, pregnant, and nursing mothers
Reproductive Behavior	White foam-like discharge from male quails when light pressure is applied to the vent region
Feed Consumption	500 g of feed up to 5 weeks of age

Advantage	Details
Hardiness	Adaptable to various environments
Housing Requirements	Does not require sophisticated housing
Space Efficiency	Requires less space for floor, feeder, and water compared to chickens and ducks
Growth and Maturity	Matures in about six weeks and reaches full production by seven weeks of age
Prolific Layers	Approximately 280 eggs annually
Disease Resistance	Resistant to many avian diseases; typically does not require vaccination

Management of Quails

Quails can be managed using a deep-litter system, a cage system, or a combination of both, but they are not suitable for free-range rearing. Proper management practices ensure optimal growth, health, and productivity of the birds. Here are the key aspects of quail management:

1. Housing Systems

- **Deep-Litter System:** Provides a natural environment with bedding material.
- **Cage System:** Efficient use of space and easier management of feed and waste.
- **Combination System:** Incorporates elements of both deep-litter and cage systems to balance benefits.

2. Space Requirements

Table 19.11: Space requirement of quail at different age

Age (weeks)	Floor space (sq. cm/bird)	Feeder space (cm/bird)	Drinker space (cm/bird)
Up to 3	75	2.0	1.0
3 to 5	100	3.5	2.0
6 to 8	125	5.0	2.5
9 and above	150	7.0	4.0

3. Temperature Management

- Maintain a brooding temperature of 35°C during the first week.
- Gradually reduce the temperature by 2.8°C every 5th day until reaching room temperature.

4. Lighting Requirements

- Provide 24 hours of light during the first two weeks of life.
- Gradually reduce to 12 hours of light starting from the 3rd week onwards.

These management practices are crucial for ensuring the health and productivity of quails throughout their development stages.

Quail Diet and Management

Quails are fed different diets according to their growth stage to meet their nutritional needs and ensure optimal health and productivity. The dietary requirements vary for starter, grower, and layer or breeder phases.

Table 19.12: Dietary nutrient requirement of quail

Nutrients	**Starter (0 to 3 weeks)**	**Grower (4 to 6 weeks)**	**Layer/breeder (7 weeks onwards)**
ME Kcal/Kg	2850	2750	2650
Protein (%)	25 to 27	22 to 24	20 to 22
Calcium (%)	1.0	0.8	3.0
Available Phosphorous (%)	0.45	0.45	0.45

Quail Management Practices

Table 19.13: Important management practices of quail

Aspect	Details
Feed Consumption	Layer quails consume approximately 25-30 g of feed daily.
Breeding Ratio	Maintain a male to female ratio of 1:1 or 1:2 for better fertility and egg production.
Debeaking	Perform debeaking between 15 to 20 days of age to prevent cannibalism.
Health Management	Quails are sturdy and typically do not require vaccination or deworming as preventive measures.

Guinea Fowl (Numida meleagris)

- **Native Region:** Guinea fowls are native to tropical West African countries but are now found worldwide.
- **Guinea Fowl Farming in India:** India has a large population of guinea fowls, ranking third after chickens and ducks.
- **Varieties in India:** Lavender, Pearl, and White are the three commonly known varieties.
- **Size and Flight:** Guinea fowls are smaller in size and can fly easily.
- **Sexing:** Females are about 20% heavier than males, primarily due to the development of their reproductive tract. Males can be identified by their larger helmet and coarser cry compared to females.

Table 19.14: Reproductive and productive Characteristics of Guinea Fowl

Characteristic	**Details**
Incubation Period	28 days (range: 26 to 28 days)
Young Ones	Called “Keets”
Growth Rate	Slower than that of chickens
Age at Sexual Maturity	28-32 weeks
Annual Egg Production	90-170 eggs per bird
Egg Characteristics	Smaller (35 to 45 g), thicker shells than chicken eggs

Characteristic	Details
Market Weight	At least 1.6 kg/bird, usually attained at 90 days of age
Dressing Yield	80%

Table 19.15: Advantages of Guinea Fowl Farming:

Advantage	Details
Adaptability	Well adapted to diverse agro-climatic conditions, particularly in arid and semi-arid regions.
Hardiness	Hardy and disease-resistant, with a unique ability to survive and thrive under sub-optimal management and feeding conditions due to their foraging habit.
Disease Resistance	Highly resistant to viral diseases, generally raised without vaccination.

Management of Guinea Fowl

Guinea fowl, due to their ability to fly, are best reared under an intensive management system. Proper space allocation, nutritional requirements, and management practices are crucial for their successful farming.

Space Requirements

Table 19.16: Space requirements of guinea fowl

Age	Floor space (sq. cm/bird)	Feeder space (cm/bird)	Drinker space (cm/bird)
Brooder (hover) space	25-50	1.5	1.25
0-4 weeks	450	2.5	1.25
4-8 weeks	720	2.5	1.25
8-12 weeks	900	3.75	2.00
>12 weeks	1350	6.25	2.50
Adult	1350-2700	10.0	2.5
Source: Wilson *et. al.*, 1997			

Table 19.17: Nutritional Requirements of guinea fowl

Nutrients	0 to 4 weeks (starter)	4 to 10 weeks	10 weeks to market	Layer / Breeder
Metabolizable Energy, Kcal/kg	3000	2800	2700	2900
Protein, %	25	24	18	18
Lysine, %	1.3	1.40	0.80	0.83
Methionine, %	0.52	0.47	0.30	0.55
Calcium, %	1.2	0.85	0.53	3.00

Available phosphorus, %	0.5	0.50	0.45	0.40
Riboflavin, mg/kg	3.40	3.40	3.00	4.00

Management Practices

Table 19.18: Management practices of guinea fowl

Aspect	**Details**
Male-Female Ratio	Maintain a ratio of 1:5 to obtain optimal fertility.
Breeder Lifespan	Breeders are usually kept for 2 or 3 seasons.
Hatching Eggs Storage	Store at 15.5-18.5°C with 70-80% relative humidity for optimal hatchability.
Brooding	Keets need proper brooding up to 4 weeks of age to prevent mortality due to chilling.
Grazing Access	Provide access to outside pens to graze by 10 weeks of age.
Market Readiness	Guinea fowls are ready for sale at 15 weeks, typically sold at 16 to 18 weeks of age.
Vaccination	Guinea fowls are hardy and generally do not need a specific vaccination program.

Turkey

Turkeys (*Meleagris gallopavo*) are primarily reared for their meat, and their farming is gaining popularity, especially in the southern parts of India. Below are some key characteristics and advantages of turkey farming:

Table 19.19: Special features of turkey

Asp	**Details**
Purpose	Rearing for meat production
Varieties in India	- Broad Breasted Bronze - Broad Breasted White - Beltsville Small White
Suitability	White turkeys are particularly well-suited for Indian conditions
ICAR Varieties	- CARI Virat (ICAR-Central Avian Research Institute, Izzatnagar) - Nandanam Turkey-I (TANUVAS, Chennai)
Sexual Dimorphism	- Males (Toms): Have many tail feathers which can be spread like a fan to attract females - Females (Turkey Hens): No such display
Sound	Called "Gobbling" (different from chickens' crowing and cackling)
Age at Sexual Maturity	28-30 weeks
Annual Egg Production	60-100 eggs per bird
Egg Weight	70-95 g

Asp	Details
Incubation Period	28 days

Table 19.20: Advantages of Turkey farming

Advantage	Details
Rearing System	Can be reared under a semi-intensive system in backyards.
Disease Resistance	More resistant to diseases compared to chickens.
Foraging Ability	Better foragers than chickens.
Meat Composition	Contains very low fat compared to meat of other avian species.
Market Demand	Higher demand during holidays such as Easter and Christmas.
Price and Health Benefits	Fetches higher prices due to low fat and cholesterol content. Considered white meat, preferred for its leanness and flavor.

Management of Turkeys

Turkeys require specific management practices to ensure their well-being and productivity. Below is a detailed overview of their management, including space requirements, feeding, and health practices.

Brooding and Rearing

- **Brooding Temperature:** Maintain at 35°C during the first week of life.
- **Intensive Rearing:** For the first 16 weeks to prevent early mortality due to feeding and drinking issues.
- **Deep Litter System:** Easier to manage and becoming popular in India.

Table 19.21: Space requirements of large turkeys on deep-litter system

Age	Floor Space (m^2/bird)	Age	Feeder Space (cm/bird)	Age	Drinker Space (cm/bird)
Brooder (hover) space	3.0 0	0-1 week	3.0	0-1 weeks	2.5
0-4 weeks	0.135	1-2 weeks	6.25	1-4 weeks	2.5
4-8 weeks	0.180	2-4 weeks	7.5	4-8 weeks	2.5
8-12 weeks	0.270	4-8 weeks	10.0	>8 weeks	3.0
>12 weeks	0.450	>8 weeks	12.5	Adult	3.5
Adult	0.720	Adult	15.0		
Source: Wilson *et. al.*, 1997					

Feeding and Health Practices

Effective feeding and health management are essential for the optimal growth and productivity of turkeys. Poults require a specific nutrient composition in their feed for healthy development, while proper health management practices help prevent diseases and ensure overall well-being. The following table outlines the nutritional requirements and recommended practices for turkeys at various stages of growth:

Age	Protein (%)	Metab-olizable Energy (Kcal/kg)	Lysine (%)	Methionine (%)	Calcium (%)	Available Phos-phorus (%)	Riboflavin (mg/kg)
0 to 4 weeks	25	3000	1.3	0.52	1.2	0.5	3.4
4 to 10 weeks	24	2800	1.40	0.47	0.85	0.50	3.4
10 weeks to market	18	2700	0.80	0.30	0.53	0.45	3.0
Layer/ Breeder	18	2900	0.83	0.55	3.00	0.40	4.00

Health Practices for Turkeys

Practice	Details
Artificial Insemination	Preferred due to the difficulty of natural mating; used to achieve maximum fertility.
Nesting	Provide nests for 20-25% of laying birds during the laying period.
Beak Trimming	Done at 3-5 weeks of age to prevent cannibalism and feather pecking.
Desnooding	Removal of the snood (dew bill) at 3 weeks of age to prevent head injuries and disease spread.
Immunization	Consider vaccinations for diseases such as RD, turkey rhinotracheitis, pox, pasteurellosis, and erysipelas.

Pigeon

Special Features of Pigeon

Pigeons, believed to be among the earliest birds domesticated by humans, are derived from the rock dove (*Columba livia*). They are celebrated for their cultural symbolism as emblems of peace, freedom, and love. In India, pigeons are cherished not only for their aesthetic value and recreational purposes but also for their economic potential. Their rearing provides income and employment opportunities, especially in rural areas. The unique combination of their manageable size, disease resistance, low maintenance costs, and the delicacy of their eggs and meat contributes to their growing popularity among both farmers and consumers. Pigeons are monogamous, with pairs forming lifelong bonds. They are notable for their distinctive breeding behaviors and their ability to thrive in specialized housing known as lofts. With a lifespan of approximately 12-15 years, pigeons continue to be a significant part of both historical and modern contexts.

Here are the notable features of pigeons:

- **Historical Significance:** Pigeons are among the earliest bird species domesticated by humans, used historically for various purposes.
- **Domesticated Subspecies:** The domestic pigeon (*Columba livia domestica*) is a subspecies derived from the rock dove, also known as the rock pigeon.
- **Symbolism:** Pigeons are often regarded as symbols of peace, freedom, and love.
- **Cultural Significance in India:** In India, pigeons are kept as ornamental birds for beautification and recreation. Hindu mythology also associates pigeons with bringing happiness to the family.
- **Economic and Social Benefits:** Pigeon rearing can provide a source of income and employment opportunities, especially for underprivileged rural communities.
- **Physical and Behavioral Traits:** Pigeons have a smaller body size, short generation interval, resistance to disease, and low maintenance cost. Their egg and meat are considered delicacies, which increases their popularity among consumers and farmers.
- **Breeding Characteristics:**
    - **Monogamous:** Pigeons are reared in pairs, with one male and one female kept together for life.
    - **Sexual Maturity:** Female pigeons reach sexual maturity at 5-6 months of age.
    - **Breeding Cycle:** They lay two eggs per breeding cycle, with a complete cycle taking around 2 months. Breeding can continue for up to 5 years.
    - **Incubation Period:** 17-18 days.
    - **Parental Care:** Both parents participate in incubation. The female incubates the eggs from late afternoon through the night, while the male takes over during the day. After hatching, both parents care for the squabs.
    - **Feeding Squabs:** Up to 10 days of age, squabs are fed "pigeon milk" or "crop milk" from the female pigeon. By around 26 days, squabs can take supplementary feed independently.
- **Housing:** Pigeons are housed in structures called lofts.
- **Lifespan:** Pigeons can live for about 12-15 years.

Breeds of Pigeons and Benefits of Pigeon Farming

Pigeons can be categorized based on their primary use, including meat production, entertainment, and homing. Each category includes specific breeds with distinct characteristics:

Breeds of Pigeons

Category	Breeds
Meat Breeds	White King, Texona, Silver King, Gola, Lokha
Entertainment Breeds	Moyurponkhi, Shirazi, Lahore, Fantail, Jacobin, Frillback, Modena, Trumpeter, Turbit, Mukhi, Giribaz, Templar, Lotal
Homing Pigeons	Racing Homer, Cher Ami, G.I. Joe

Benefits of Pigeon Farming

Benefit	Details
Docile and Easy to Handle	Pigeons are gentle and manageable, making them easy to care for.
Shorter Generation Interval	Approximately 2 months per breeding cycle, allowing for up to 12 squabs per year per pair.
Minimal Housing Requirements	Can be reared in home yards or rooftops without sophisticated housing.
Low Feeding Costs	Pigeons collect their own feed, minimizing feeding expenses.
Quick Maturation	Squabs are ready for consumption within 3 to 4 weeks of age.
Nutritional Value	Squab meat is lean, digestible, and rich in proteins, minerals, and vitamins, suitable for patients and elderly.
Entertainment Value	Observing pigeons provides pleasure and entertainment.
Good Returns on Investment	Requires minimal investment with potentially high returns in a short period.
Disease Resistance	Generally resistant to common avian diseases.
Utilization of Feathers	Feathers can be used to make various types of toys.
Environmental Benefits	Pigeons help control insect populations, contributing to environmental health.

Emu

The emu(*Dromaius novaehollandiae*), a large flightless bird native to Australia, is the third-largest bird in the world, following the ostrich and cassowary. Known as the "million-dollar bird," emus have become a valuable resource in various industries due to their unique attributes.

Special Features of Emu

Feature	Details
Origin	Australia
Size	Third largest bird in the world, 1.5-1.8 meters tall, weighing 45-60 kg
Commercial Farming in India	Began in 1996 with imports from the USA; initially undertaken by 'Vijaya Ratites,' later sold to 'Flightless Birds of India' (FBI) in 1997
Economic Value	Emu fat is used for oil with dietary, therapeutic (anti-inflammatory), and cosmetic benefits.
Cosmetic Value	Emu oil is preferred over mineral oil for its better skin penetration.
Leather and Feathers	Emu leather is used in designer apparel, boots, wallets, and accessories; feathers are used in fashion, art, and crafts.
Egg Production	Average annual egg production is 25 eggs, with each egg weighing about 575 grams.
Meat Yield	An adult emu yields approximately 15 kg of boneless meat, 10 kg of body fat, 0.75 square meter of skin, and two leg skins.
Dressing Yield	Up to 70%
Reproductive Longevity	Can reproduce for up to 25 years
Life Span	25-30 years
Age at Sexual Maturity	52 weeks
Incubation Period	52-55 days

Emu farming offers diverse benefits, from meat and leather to oil and feathers, making it a valuable enterprise with a range of applications in various industries.

Management of Emu

Emus are managed under a semi-intensive system, requiring specific space and care considerations throughout their life stages. An overview of their management practices is depicted below:

Table 19.22: Space requirements for Emu

Age	Floor Space (m^2/bird)	Feeder Space (cm/bird)	Drinker Space (cm/bird)
Brooder (hover) space	0.135	10	15
0-4 weeks	0.72	15	15
4-8 weeks	1.35	22.5	15
8-12 weeks	2.70	22.5	15
>12 weeks	5.40	22.5	15
Adult	0.04-0.12*	22.5	15
*Hectare for 2 to 4 birds		Source: Wilson *et. al.*, 1997	

Management practices for Emu

Aspect	Details
Housing	Emus are reared in pairs with a minimum space of 18m × 9m for run space and 2.4m × 2.4m for shelter.
Sexing	Done at day-old through feather sexing, vent sexing, and sound differentiation on maturity.
Breeding Season	October to February (winter season) in India.
Incubation	Males incubate eggs for 52 to 55 days without food or water; females breed with other partners.
Chick Care	Males care for chicks post-hatching. Brooding temperatures: 90°F for the first 10 days, 85°F till 3-4 weeks. Chicks need water but get nourishment from yolk for 2-3 days.
Diet	Consists of fruits, flowers, insects, seeds, green vegetation, and caterpillars.
Feed Intake	Adults consume 1.4 to 1.5 kg of feed and drink 6 to 10 liters of water daily.
Commercial Feed Types	- **Chick Starter**: Up to 2-3 months of age. - **Grower**: Up to 8 months of age. - **Finisher**: Until 14-16 months of age. - **Breeder**: From 16 months onwards. - **Maintenance**: After completion of lay until next breeding season.

The suggested nutrient requirements of emu birds are as follows:

Table 19.23: Nutrient requirement of emu

Nutrients	Starter	Grower	Finisher	Breeder	Maintenance
ME (kcal/kg)	2700	2600	2600	2600	2400
Crude Protein (%)	20	18	16	20	15
Lysine (%)	1.0	0.8	0.7	0.9	0.63
Methionine (%)	0.45	0.4	0.35	0.40	0.25
Calcium (%)	1.5	1.5	1.5	2.50	1.6
Available phosphorus (%)	0.55	0.5	0.40	0.4	0.4
(Source: Reddy, 2004, Scheideler, 1997)					

- Emus are resistant to most diseases and generally do not require vaccination.
- Ivermectin can be administered at 1-month intervals, starting at 1 month of age, to prevent external and internal worms.

OSTRICH (*Srruthio camelus*)

Ostrich farming has gained prominence as a lucrative venture due to the unique qualities and diverse products derived from ostriches (*Struthio camelus*). Native to sub-Saharan Africa, ostriches are the largest and fastest flightless birds in the world, known for their impressive size and distinctive features.

With males weighing between 100-130 kg and standing up to 9 feet tall, these birds are highly valued not only for their meat but also for their feathers, skin, and oil. The farming of ostriches is increasingly seen as a sustainable agricultural practice, offering economic benefits through the production of high-quality leather, feather products, and oil used in cosmetics and food products. Their adaptability to various climates and long productive lifespan of up to 42 years make them an attractive option for farmers looking to diversify their agricultural enterprises. As the demand for ostrich products continues to rise, ostrich farming presents opportunities for both traditional and innovative uses of these remarkable birds.

General Information on Ostriches

Characteristic	Details
Native Region	Sub-Saharan Africa
Size	7-9 feet in height
Adult Male Weight	100-130 kg
Adult Female Weight	90-110 kg
Breeding Age	2-3 years
Breeding Duration	Up to 20 years
Annual Egg Production	About 40 eggs
Egg Weight	1100-1600 g
Incubation Period	About 42 days
Life Span	40-70 years
Economic Productive Period	Up to 42 years
Skin Uses	Luxury items (boots, handbags, billfolds)
Feather Uses	Cleaning fine machinery
Oil Uses	Moisturizers, body lotion, soap, lip balm; used in foods due to low cholesterol

Management of Ostriches

Ostriches are versatile birds capable of thriving in a range of climates, provided they receive appropriate care and management. During winter months, they need housing with access to outdoor exercise to maintain their health and well-being. Effective fencing is crucial for older juveniles and adults, requiring at least 5 feet in height and constructed with five to seven strands of smooth, barbless wire to ensure safety and containment.

Breeding management is optimized with a flock ratio of 1 male to 2 females, fostering better fertility. Natural incubation involves males incubating eggs at night and females during the day, while artificial incubation requires precise conditions: eggs should be stored at 55-65°F with 75% relative humidity, and incubated at a constant 37.5°C.

Brooding practices are essential for reducing early chick mortality. Initially, the brooding temperature should be maintained at 31.1 to 33°C, gradually decreasing to 23.5°C by 3 to 8 weeks of age. Chicks can be introduced to outdoor ranges by 6 to 8 weeks, but must be sheltered at night. By 4 months, they are more resilient and can range outside with fewer risks.

Shelter and shade are vital for protecting ostriches and their feed from inclement weather. The pen floor should be rough to prevent "spraddled legs" in chicks, a common condition caused by slick surfaces or improper litter materials. Avoid using smooth materials such as newspaper or plastic in the pen, as they can exacerbate this issue and lead to significant mortality among young birds.

Table Management

Management Aspect	Details
Climate Adaptation	Can adapt to most climates; needs housing in winter with outdoor access.
Fencing Requirements	At least 5 feet high with 5-7 strands of smooth, barbless wire.
Breeding Ratio	Maintain a 1:2 (trio) ratio of males to females for better fertility.
Natural Incubation	Male incubates eggs at night, female during the day.
Artificial Incubation Conditions	Eggs stored at 55-65°F with 75% humidity; incubated at 37.5°C.
Brooding Temperature	31.1-33°C for the first two weeks; gradually reduce to 23.5°C by 3-8 weeks.
Outdoor Ranging	Introduce to range by 6-8 weeks; provide shelter at night.
Hardiness	Chicks are hardy by 4 months and can range outside safely.
Shelter and Shade	Necessary to protect birds and feed from weather.
Floor and Litter Management	Use rough floor surfaces; avoid slick materials like newspaper or plastic.

Table 19.24: Suggested space requirements for trio (1+2):

Category	Indoor space	Outdoor space
1-21 Days	2 sq.ft/bird	10-15 sq.ft /bird
22-90 Days	30sq.ft/bird	30 sq.ft/bird
90-300 Days	300sq. ft/bird	2000sq.ft/bird
Breeder/Selection	No indoor space	1500-2000 sq.ft/bird
12 Months and Older	500 sq.ft/bird	2000 sq.ft/bird
		Source: Abbas *et. al.,* 2018

Feeding and Health Management of Ostriches

Ostriches are adaptable grazers and browsers, thriving on a varied diet that includes grass, berries, succulents, seeds, and leaves from trees and bushes.

However, baby ostrich chicks often face issues with eating and drinking, leading to high early mortality rates. To address this, older chicks (1-3 weeks old) or indigenous chicks can be placed with younger chicks to encourage feeding behavior. Continuous light and access to starter feed are essential for chicks during the first three weeks, after which night lighting can be discontinued.

Access to clean, potable water is crucial at all times. Feeders and waterers should be open types and adjustable to chest height for ease of use. It is vital to avoid offering moldy, musty, wet, or spoiled feeds to prevent health issues such as botulism or intestinal problems.

The recommended nutrient requirements of ostrich are as follows:

Table 19.24: Recommended nutrient requirement of ostrich

Nutrients	**Starter (0 to 8 weeks)**	**Grower (9 weeks to 17 months)**	**Breeder (18 months onwards)**
ME (kcal/kg)	2600	2500	2500
Crude Protein (%)	18	18	24
Lysine (%)	1.0	0.85	1.0
Methionine (%)	0.36	0.36	0.36
Calcium (%)	1.35	1.35	2.4
Available phosphorus (%)	0.72	0.64	0.70
			Source: Reddy, 2005

Ostriches are generally resistant to most diseases, reducing the need for vaccinations. However, to prevent external and internal worms, Ivermectin should be administered at one-month intervals starting from one month of age.

20

Marketing of Poultry and Poultry Products

Rafiqul Islam and Mihir Sarma

Marketing of Poultry and Poultry Products

Marketing involves the exchange of produce for an agreed sum of money and is a critical commercial process that encompasses promoting, selling, and distributing products. At its core, marketing is about understanding customer needs and providing products that meet these needs profitably. It is an essential business function that focuses on customer satisfaction and business growth.

Objectives of Marketing

1. **Employment Generation:** Marketing creates gainful employment opportunities for millions, thereby increasing income levels.
2. **Demand Enhancement:** It aims to boost the demand for poultry products, which in turn generates more employment opportunities in rural areas.
3. **Improved Standards of Living:** By providing essential nutrients like amino acids, fatty acids, vitamins, and minerals through poultry products, marketing contributes to the better health and standard of living of poultry farmers.
4. **Efficient Supply:** Ensures that poultry products are available at the right time, place, quantity, and price.
5. **Organized Marketing System:** Contributes to improved societal living standards by identifying and meeting the needs of the community.

Various Activities Involved in Marketing

- **Collection:** Gathering poultry products from producers.
- **Evaluation:** Assessing the quality and value of poultry products.
- **Dissemination of Marketing Information:** Sharing relevant market information with stakeholders.
- **Planning & Scheduling of Production:** Organizing production schedules to meet market demand.

- **Forming Contacts:** Establishing relationships between buyers and sellers.
- **Constant Improvement:** Enhancing all post-harvest activities to ensure product quality.
- **Coordinating Inputs:** Managing inputs like transport, processing, storage, credit, and healthcare to optimize the supply chain.

Status of Export of Poultry and Poultry Products in India

India's role in the global poultry market is relatively modest, but it has made significant strides in certain areas. Here's an overview of India's current status in poultry exports:

- **Global Trade Share:** India's share of the world trade in poultry and poultry products remains small.
- **Dried Egg Exports:** India leads the world in the export of dried eggs, according to FAO data from 2007.
- **Duck Exports:** India ranks 8th globally in duck exports.
- **Major Export Products:** India exports a variety of poultry products including live poultry, hatching eggs, table eggs, egg powder, frozen eggs, poultry meat, and specific pathogen free (SPF) eggs.
- **Export Statistics (2022-23):** According to APEDA, India exported 664,753.46 MT of poultry products valued at Rs. 1,081.62 Crores (approximately 134.04 USD Million) during the fiscal year 2022-23.
- **Major Export Destinations:** The primary markets for Indian poultry products include Oman, Indonesia, Maldives, United Arab Emirates, and Japan.

Marketing of Eggs

The marketing of eggs encompasses the entire process of moving eggs from producers to consumers, ensuring that these products reach the market efficiently and effectively. Eggs are marketed in various forms, including whole eggs, processed eggs, and specialized egg products, catering to diverse consumer needs. Price variability is a common feature in the egg market, with prices fluctuating based on factors such as geographic location and seasonal changes. The primary objective of egg marketing is to ensure that high-quality eggs are delivered to consumers, maintaining both the freshness of the product and consumer satisfaction.

Organizations Involved in Egg Marketing in India

National Egg Coordination Committee (NECC)

Aspect	**Details**
Formation	Established on May 14, 1982, by Dr. B.V. Rao
Membership	Over 25,000 poultry farmers
Motto	"My egg, my price, my life"
Significance	The largest association of poultry farmers globally
Unique Feature	Provides official notified prices to farmers regardless of size or location
Recognition	Acknowledged by state and central policymakers as a key representative body for the poultry industry

Role of NECC

Role	Function	Objective
Market Intervention	NECC intervenes in the egg market to stabilize prices during periods of volatility. This can involve direct action to influence supply and demand or coordinate with stakeholders to manage market fluctuations.	To prevent extreme price variations that could negatively impact both producers and consumers.
Price Support Operations	NECC supports prices by setting minimum prices for eggs, ensuring that producers receive fair compensation for their products. This can involve buying surplus eggs or providing financial support.	To ensure that egg prices remain stable and fair, providing financial security for producers.
Egg Promotion Campaigns	NECC conducts promotional activities to increase the demand for eggs. This includes advertising, public relations, and educational campaigns to highlight the benefits of egg consumption.	To boost consumer demand and expand the market for eggs, leading to increased sales and profitability.
Consumer Education	NECC provides information to consumers about the nutritional benefits and quality of eggs. This can involve educational programs, informational materials, and outreach initiatives.	To increase consumer awareness and encourage higher egg consumption by educating them about the benefits.
Market Research	NECC conducts research to gather data on egg production, consumption trends, and market conditions. This research helps in making informed decisions and strategies for the industry.	To understand market dynamics and trends, aiding in better decision-making and strategic planning for the poultry sector.
Rural Market Development	NECC focuses on developing rural markets by improving infrastructure and providing support to poultry farmers in rural areas. This includes facilitating access to markets and resources.	To enhance market access and support the growth of poultry farming in rural areas, improving livelihoods and economic conditions.
Liaison with Government on Industry Issues	NECC engages with government bodies to address issues affecting the poultry industry. This includes advocating for policies and regulations that benefit the industry.	To represent the interests of poultry farmers and ensure that government policies support the growth and stability of the poultry sector.
Operates on Cooperative Principles	NECC operates based on cooperative principles, emphasizing collective decision-making and voluntary contributions from its members. It does not seek profit but focuses on the welfare of its members.	To foster a cooperative environment where members work together to achieve common goals and support each other

Two strategies are taken by the NECC to declare and maintain the prices of eggs

- **Egg Promotion Campaigns:** To increase market size and demand.
- **Market Intervention:** To stabilize egg prices.

Agro-Corpex India Limited (ACIL)

- **Ownership:** Public limited company, fully owned and managed by poultry farmers.
- **Affiliations:** Associated with Bharat Egg Producers' Association (BEPA), which supports the export of shelled eggs, promotes eggs through media, and sponsors activities to boost poultry consumption.

The marketing of eggs in India is facilitated by major organizations like NECC and ACIL, which work to stabilize prices, promote consumption, and support poultry farmers. These bodies play a crucial role in ensuring the efficient distribution and marketing of eggs, contributing to both the economic well-being of farmers and the availability of quality eggs to consumers.

National Agricultural Co-operative Marketing Federation of India (NAFED)

The National Agricultural Co-operative Marketing Federation of India (NAFED) plays a pivotal role in the marketing of eggs across various regions in India. NAFED's responsibilities include managing egg supplies in major urban and industrial areas, providing support prices to poultry farmers during market downturns, and handling surplus stocks through its cold storage facilities. The following table details NAFED's involvement and its collaborative efforts with the National Egg Coordination Committee (NECC) to stabilize the egg market.

Aspect	Details
Role in Egg Marketing	NAFED manages egg marketing in New Delhi and extends to major terminal markets in Mumbai, Chennai, Kolkata, Hyderabad, and other industrial areas.
Support Price	Announcements of support prices for eggs during periods of market slumps to assist small poultry farmers.
Cold Storage	Operates its own cold storage facilities to manage surplus eggs received during peak seasons.
Collaboration with NECC	NAFED's activities are based on recommendations from NECC, and any financial losses due to these interventions are shared by the government and NECC.

Marketing Channels for Eggs

Marketing channels are crucial in determining how eggs move from producers to consumers. These channels vary in complexity and efficiency, affecting both the cost and the final price of eggs. Understanding these channels helps in identifying the benefits and drawbacks of each route, from direct sales to cooperative marketing. The table below outlines the different marketing channels available for eggs, illustrating the various routes through which eggs are distributed. Broadly there are 4 marketing channels:

Sl. No.	Channel	Description
1	Direct Marketing	Producer sells eggs directly to consumers, eliminating intermediaries. This benefits both the producer and the consumer by reducing costs and improving prices.
2	Indirect Marketing	Eggs move from the producer to the consumer via retailers. This channel involves intermediaries who handle the distribution and sale of eggs.
3	Integrated Marketing	Eggs are sold through collectors or commission agents who facilitate the movement from producers to consumers. This channel involves several intermediaries.
4	Co-operative Marketing	Eggs are marketed through cooperative societies. Farmers benefit from additional services like access to cheap feed, medicines, technical advice, and sometimes day-old chicks at lower prices.

Price Spread

The price spread refers to the difference between the cost of producing eggs and the retail price at which they are sold. This spread can be significantly influenced by the number of intermediaries involved in the marketing channels. Understanding the price spread helps in evaluating the efficiency of different marketing routes and their impact on both producers and consumers. The following table illustrates how the price spread can vary with different marketing channels.

Aspect	Details
Price Spread	The difference between the cost of production and the retail price of eggs increases with the number of intermediaries involved in the marketing channel.

Challenges of Egg Marketing

The marketing of eggs in India faces several challenges that impact the quality and efficiency of distribution. Eggs are often transported in open conditions and un-refrigerated vehicles, exposing them to varying temperatures and seasonal agro-climatic conditions. This exposure significantly limits their shelf life-ranging from 11-14 days in summer to 18-20 days in winter. Additionally, eggs are commonly sold as a commodity in local shops and *kirana* stores, which may not always ensure optimal handling and storage. Following challenges highlight the need for improvements in the egg marketing infrastructure to enhance product quality and consumer satisfaction.By addressing these challenges and implementing the suggested strategies, the efficiency and effectiveness of egg marketing in India can be significantly improved.

Suggestions for Successful Egg Marketing

To address the challenges in egg marketing and improve the overall efficiency of the supply chain, several strategies can be implemented:

1. **Formation of Cooperative Societies:** Encouraging the establishment of cooperative societies can streamline egg production and distribution, ensuring better handling and marketing practices.
2. **Grading and Pricing:** Adoption of grading standards as per the Bureau of Indian Standards (BIS) should be promoted, with pricing based on the quality grades to ensure fairness and transparency.
3. **Cold Storage Facilities:** Creating and maintaining cold storage facilities will help in reducing spoilage and extending the shelf life of eggs, especially during fluctuations in supply and demand.
4. **Improved Packaging and Transportation:** Ensuring proper care during packaging and transportation is essential to maintain egg quality and prevent damage.
5. **Sales Promotion and Consumer Education:** Implementing vigorous campaigns to promote egg sales and educate consumers about the nutritional benefits of eggs can drive demand & increase market acceptance.

Challenges of Marketing Poultry Meat

The marketing of poultry meat in India faces several significant challenges that impact both producers and consumers. These challenges arise from various factors including market volatility, inefficient distribution channels, and seasonal supply-demand imbalances. Understanding these issues is crucial for developing strategies to improve the marketing and overall efficiency of the poultry meat sector. Below is a summary of the key challenges:

Challenge	Description
Market Range	Poultry meat is marketed from street corner live bird slaughterhouses to highly sophisticated, ISO-certified facilities offering ready-to-eat products.
Price Volatility	Prices fluctuate widely based on daily demand and supply, with short-term surpluses leading to significant price swings.

Lack of Coordinated Channels	There is no coordinated marketing channel for poultry meat, leading to inefficiencies in the supply chain.
Dependence on Traditional Traders	Small and medium farmers often rely on traditional traders for marketing, who may exploit them.
Economic Losses Due to Overproduction	Overproduction compared to market demand can result in substantial economic losses for farmers.
Exploitation by Middlemen	Middlemen frequently exploit poultry farmers, exacerbating market inefficiencies.
Seasonal Supply Fluctuations	Supply and demand vary seasonally, with summer supply often below demand and winter supply exceeding demand, affected by growth rates and consumer habits.
Reduced Consumption During Festivals	Non-vegetarian consumption drops during festival months such as Shravan, Ganesh Chaturthi, and Navaratri, impacting overall demand.

Opportunities for Marketing Poultry Products

The marketing of poultry products presents several promising opportunities for growth and expansion. Identifying and leveraging these opportunities can help meet the increasing demand and enhance the overall market reach. Here's a look at the key opportunities in the poultry sector:

Opportunity	**Description**
Rural Market Expansion	Although eggs and meat are widely available in urban and semi-urban areas, rural areas still have low availability. There is significant potential to increase market penetration in these areas.
Export Potential	There is an opportunity to export poultry products, such as eggs and meat, to the Middle East and European countries, expanding market reach and boosting revenue.
Inclusion in Mid-Day Meal Scheme	Incorporating eggs into the Mid-day Meal Scheme across all states can increase consumption and improve the nutritional status of underprivileged students. Eggs, being a balanced and non-adulterated food item, are an ideal choice for this scheme.

Current Broiler Market Size in India

The current market dynamics of broiler poultry in India reflect varied consumer preferences and market segmentation:

Market Segment	**Percentage of Market Share**
Branded Chicken and Chicken Products	Less than 1%
Chilled or Frozen Chicken	4-5%
Live Bird Sales in Wet Market	95%

21

Water Quality and Its Management in Poultry Production

Pankaj Deka and Rafiqul Islam

Water is a critical and essential nutrient in poultry production, necessary in greater amounts than any other nutrient. It plays a vital role in various physiological processes such as digestion, metabolism, nutrient transportation, enzymatic and chemical reactions, regulating body temperature, and lubricating joints and organs. Water deprivation can have severe consequences on poultry health, impacting growth, egg production, and even leading to increased mortality if prolonged. Therefore, providing cool, clean water that is free from contaminants is crucial for maintaining poultry health and optimizing farm profitability.

Water Consumption in Poultry

Water consumption in poultry varies under different conditions. Generally, under thermo-neutral conditions, birds will consume approximately twice the amount of water as the amount of feed. However, water intake is influenced by several factors, including environmental temperature, relative humidity, dietary salt and protein levels, the productivity of the birds (growth rate or egg production), and the bird's ability to reabsorb water in the kidneys. In poultry houses, water consumption tends to be higher in areas with more birds and higher ambient temperatures. Studies indicate that birds prefer water at about 10°C; when water temperatures exceed 27°C, both water intake and daily weight gain are significantly reduced.

Ensuring proper water quality and managing water consumption are essential for maintaining the health and productivity of poultry.

Water Consumption in Poultry Production

Water consumption in poultry varies depending on the production stage, environmental conditions, and bird type. The tables below provide a detailed overview of the typical water consumption rates for layer chickens and broilers under different conditions.

Table 21.1: Typical water consumption of layer chicken at 21°C

Production stage	Age or rate of production	Water consumption (litres) per 1000 birds
Pullet	4 weeks	100
	12 weeks	160
	18 weeks	200
Layer hens	50%	220
	90%	270

This table illustrates how water consumption increases as pullets mature and as layer hens reach higher production rates.

Table 21.2: Water consumption (litres) per 1000 of broiler at different temperatures

Age (weeks)	10.0°C	21.1°C	32.2°C	37.8°C
1	30	30	34	38
2	45	61	98	182
3	72	95	197	360
4	98	133	273	492
5	133	174	356	644
6	163	216	416	757
7	189	254	462	863

This table shows how water consumption increases with both age and environmental temperature, highlighting the need for careful water management in varying climatic conditions.

Common poultry diseases transmitted through water

Drinking water is a crucial factor in the transmission of various infectious diseases in poultry. Contaminated water can serve as a medium for spreading bacterial, viral, and protozoan diseases, which can significantly impact poultry health and production. The table below outlines some of the most common poultry diseases transmitted through water.

Table 21.3: Common infectious diseases transmitted through water

Bacterial Diseases	Viral Diseases	Protozoan Diseases
Chronic Respiratory Disease (CRD)	Ranikhet Disease (Newcastle Disease)	Coccidiosis
Colibacillosis (E. coli Infection)	Avian Influenza	Histomoniasis (Blackhead Disease)
Fowl Cholera	Marek's Disease	
Fowl Typhoid	Avian Encephalomyelitis	

Pullorum Disease (Salmonella Pullorum)	Infectious Bursal Disease (Gumboro)	
Infectious Coryza	Infectious Bronchitis	
Salmonellosis	Avian Pox	
Necrotic Enteritis	Infectious Laryngotracheitis	

Standards of water quality for poultry

Table 21.4: Maximum acceptable levels of contaminants in drinking water

Contaminant or characteristics level	Average level	Maximum acceptable level	Remarks
Bacteria: 1. Total bacteria 2. Coliform bacteria	 0/ml 0/ml	 100 cfu/ml 50cfu/ml	 0/ml desirable 0/ml desirable
Colour	Colourless	-	-
Nitrogen compounds 1. Nitrate 2. Nitrite	 2 ppm 0.4 ppm	 20 ppm 4 ppm	Performance effected at <50 ppm of nitrate; nitrite is 10 times more toxic than nitrate
pH	6.0 to 6.8	-	A pH less than 6.0 is not desirable. Levels below 6.3 may degradeperformances
Total hardness	60-189 ppm	-	Hardness below 60 is too soft while above 180 is too hard
Total dissolved solids	<1000 ppm	-	No serious burden in any class of poultry
Calcium	60 ppm	100 ppm	Binds with tetracycline, precipitate in water system
Magnesium	14 ppm	125 ppm	Wet droppings, interfere with nutrient absorption specially in presence of sulphate
Chloride	14 ppm	250 ppm	If Na is high, low chloride is detrimental; high NaCl may reduce performance and reduce shell quality
Sodium	32 ppm	50 ppm	If sulphate or chloride is high, performance effected
Sulfate	125 ppm	250 ppm	Laxative effect with magnesium, fast bleeding and oedema
Iron	0.2 ppm	0.3 ppm	Precipitate clogs water systems
Lead	-	0.02 ppm	Kidney failure, nervous disorder
Cadmium	-	0.01 ppm	Kidney failure
Source: Poultry Year Book, 2003-04			

Measures to improve water quality in poultry production

Measure	Description	Application/Examples
Chlorination	A widely used bactericidal method for disinfecting drinking water in poultry farms.	Bleaching powder (calcium hypochlorite) is commonly used to effectively kill harmful bacteria and prevent diseases.
Acidification	Lowers the pH of drinking water, inhibiting microbial growth.	Propionic, formic, peracetic, and acetic acids are used; higher concentrations should be avoided to prevent equipment damage.
Amenities and Cleaning	Prevents biofilm formation in water supply systems.	Concentrated acidifiers and specific cleaning chemicals are used to reduce biofilm growth and maintain clean water lines.
Plant-Based Extracts	Utilizes biocidal properties of plant extracts to control infections in water.	Cimerol ring-containing extracts are effective against bacteria like Salmonella, Pseudomonas, Clostridium, and E. coli.
Physical Methods	Improves water quality by removing contaminants and balancing chemical parameters.	Techniques like reverse osmosis, filtration, and flocculation are used to treat water, ensuring it meets poultry standards.

Water Management Tips for Poultry Production

1. Conduct Regular Water Testing

- Regular testing of well water on each farm is crucial. Water quality can fluctuate during periods of heavy rain or drought, which can impact water availability and quality. Conducting additional tests during these times ensures that water lines continue to deliver sufficient water for both the birds and the cooling systems, maintaining optimal health and performance.

2. Change Filters Regularly

- Replace filters consistently to prevent sediment and particulates from causing leaks in water nipples, which can degrade litter quality. Clogged filters restrict water flow to drinkers and cooling systems, leading to inadequate water supply. For water sources with high iron content or other challenges, simple cartridge filters may not suffice, and alternative water treatments should be considered.

3. Flush Water Lines Regularly

- Perform high-pressure flushing of water lines between each flock to remove any residual contaminants. This is especially important after administering supplements through medicators, such as vaccines, medications, vitamins, or electrolytes, to prevent build-up and ensure clean water delivery.

4. Plan Water Treatment Carefully

- Before initiating any water treatment or sanitation programs, consult with a veterinarian. This ensures that treatments do not interact negatively with existing water contaminants, which could result in clogging or other issues within the water system. Proper planning prevents potential disruptions and maintains water quality.

Index

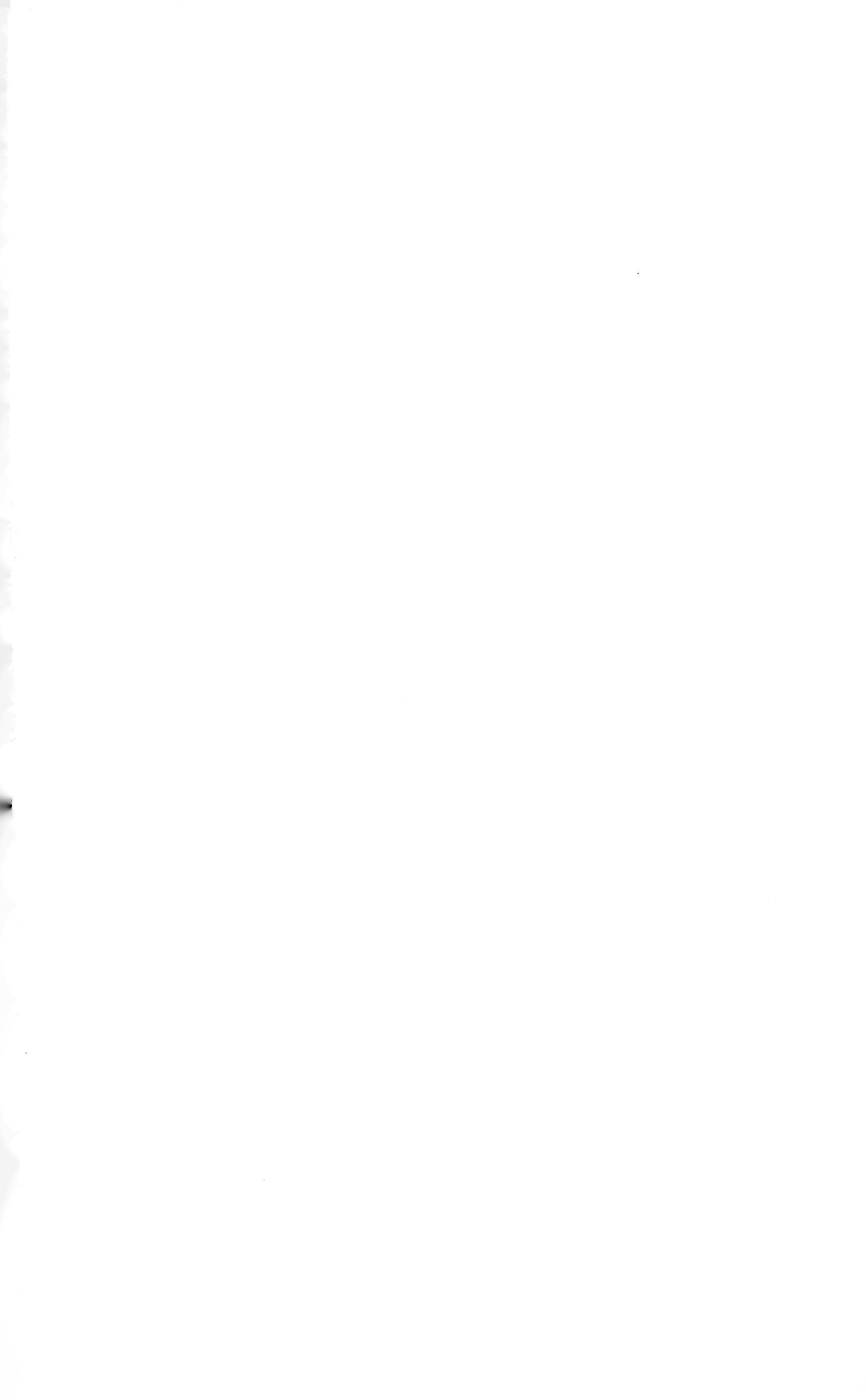